Feel Good Again

Feel Good Again

Coping with the Emotions of Illness

Stephen A. Green, M.D.,
and the Editors of
Consumer Reports Books

CONSUMERS UNION   MOUNT VERNON, NEW YORK

The editors of Consumer Reports Books give special thanks to
Peter Bejger for his help in developing the text of this book.

The ideas, procedures, and suggestions contained in this book are
not intended to replace the services of a physician. All matters regarding your health require medical supervision, and you should
consult a physician before adopting the procedures in this book.
Any application of the treatments set forth herein are at the reader's discretion, and neither the authors nor the publisher assumes
any responsibility or liability therefor.

The cases and examples cited in this book are based on actual
situations and real people. Names and identifying details have
been changed to protect privacy.

Library of Congress Cataloging-in-Publication Data
Green, Stephen A., 1945–
Feel good again: coping with the emotions of illness / Stephen A.
Green and the editors of Consumer Reports Books.
    p. cm.
ISBN 0-89043-413-1 ISBN 0-89043-300-3 (pbk.)
1. Medicine and psychology. 2. Sick—Psychology. 3. Adjustment
(Psychology) I. Consumer Reports Books. II. Title.
R726.5.G73   1990
616'.001'9—dc20   90-35584
                                                            CIP

Design by Paula R. Szafranski

First printing, September 1990
Manufactured in the United States of America

Consumer Reports Books

Feel Good Again is a Consumer Reports Book published by Consumers Union, the nonprofit organization that publishes *Consumer Reports*, the monthly magazine of test reports, product Ratings, and buying guidance. Established in 1936, Consumers Union is chartered under the Not-for-Profit Corporation Law of the State of New York.

The purposes of Consumers Union, as stated in its charter, are to provide consumers with information and counsel on consumer goods and services, to give information on all matters relating to the expenditure of the family income, and to initiate and to cooperate with individual and group efforts seeking to create and maintain decent living standards.

For Madeleine, Jessica, and Julia

Contents

Acknowledgments

The publication of any book is such a complicated and arduous process, involving so many people, that I find it impossible to properly acknowledge the many whose encouragement, support, and hard work combined to produce this volume. However, I want to extend my particular appreciation to Jill Zaklow, for excellent substantive and editorial contributions; to Richard Suzman, whose technical expertise liberated text from uncooperative floppy disks; and to Julia, the consummate "spellchecker."

A final word of gratitude to those whose energy and empathy have been central to my development as a physician. My interest in psychiatry began when I was a student of Dr. Vernon Sharp, and it solidified during my medical internship under the guidance and friendship of Dr. Don R. Lipsitt. The instruction I received during my psychiatric residency training from faculty and colleagues—particularly Drs. Elvin Semrad, Steven Sharfstein, and Sheldon Roth—has been invaluable over the years. Those who taught me best possessed a common characteristic, a basic respect for patients as human beings with distinctive fears, wishes, and needs in health and illness.

Feel Good Again

Introduction

I met John Wilson during my third year of medical school. He was admitted to the hospital because of progressive weakness and fatigue and was subsequently diagnosed with a debilitating case of tuberculosis. Although he responded well to treatment, Mr. Wilson seemed neither relieved nor grateful. He became increasingly argumentative with the staff and periodically refused to take his medication. Annoyed by this behavior, his caretakers steadily distanced themselves from him. This further complicated his treatment, for he threatened to leave the hospital against medical advice because he believed that no one was taking care of him. The potential effect on his future health was obviously grave.

Mr. Wilson's growing reputation as "the ward's problem patient" eventually prompted his physician to request a psychiatric consultation. During this meeting, the patient recounted his history intelligently, but with an obvious sadness. When asked about his mood, he became somewhat suspicious and wary of the psychiatrist's motivations, because few physicians had ever expressed an

1

interest in his emotional state. However, with gentle, persistent prodding, he responded to the question.

The patient reported that he had recently moved to New York City, having lived all his life in the South, and felt isolated and frightened there. His failing strength prevented him from working, and his growing concern about being able to provide for himself prompted him to seek medical attention. He recognized his recent improvement but remained pessimistic about the future, anticipating frequent relapses and progressive debility. He believed his disease would eventually become untreatable and that he would die young, a fear aggravated by a considerable shame about his morbid preoccupations. He also resented the aloofness of his physicians, experiencing them as emotionally unavailable whenever he attempted to discuss concerns about his future health.

The psychiatrist suggested that separation from the support of family and friends would heighten anyone's concern about the ability to be self-sufficient. Moreover, it might cause one to crave added attention from medical personnel. At this point, the patient began to sob. After several minutes he composed himself, made no apologies for his tears, and proceeded to talk about himself in an animated fashion. He continued, essentially uninterrupted, for the remainder of the meeting. As he spoke, his spirits lifted; his relief was palpable.

Observing this interview was an indelible experience in my early training, one that propelled me toward the future practice of psychiatry. The patient's treatment had successfully addressed physical symptoms while neglecting his emotional needs. His caretakers had failed to evaluate and attend to powerful, debilitating feelings precipitated by his illness, and consequently, despite physical improvement, his overall ability to function remained significantly impaired. However, a frank discussion with a psychiatrist allowed the necessary attention to his mind, as well as his body. I had witnessed an intimate interaction between two individuals in which mutual honesty enabled the patient to gain a needed perspective on the emotions stirred by his illness. A physician had helped him merely by talking with him, or, more precisely, by carefully listening to him and communicating back an empathic and accurate understanding of his plight. The patient felt less isolated, and thus less handicapped by the powerful emotions he had been unable to contend with by himself. Responding to the consultant's support, he was finally able to explore the feelings unleashed by his illness, which diminished his fear of becoming overwhelmed by them. He began a dramatic improvement in his overall condition.

Mr. Wilson's case illustrates a fundamental shortcoming of current health care, one that can seriously compromise the welfare of any patient—namely, an institutionalized dichotomy that separates medical illness from issues of the mind. Many health providers define a disease exclusively in terms of its physical manifestations and consequently treat only the obvious physical symptoms. However, there is extensive scientific evidence that highlights the inextricable link between mind and body, proving that *patients' emotions both affect, and are affected by, medical illness.*

The influence of specific emotional states on physical well-being is well-established. Depression, for example, is associated with a higher incidence of fatal illness. This phenomenon was demonstrated in classic medical studies of widows and of hospitalized infants deprived of sufficient nurturing during this crucial period of their development. An equally important facet of mind-body interaction concerns the impact of physical illness on emotions. All medical illness—whether minor or serious, acute or chronic, treatable or terminal—produces a distinct emotional reaction that is an integral part of the particular disease. Patients regularly experience a gamut of feelings, such as anger, anxiety, depression, and helplessness, throughout the course of an illness.

Despite these findings, many health providers frequently ignore patients' feelings and treat the *disease*, as opposed to the *human being*. The negative effects of this approach are several. First, it interferes with a patient's attempts to deal with the painful and distressing emotions brought on by the illness. This often causes considerable increase in the intensity of those feelings, producing, for example, debilitating degrees of anxiety or depression that can easily impede the overall ability to cope with the stress of ill health. Second, as with John Wilson, it can undermine the necessary therapeutic relationship between patient and medical personnel. Third, it may have the insidious effect of indirectly communicating to patient and family that the expression of emotions is unnecessary and perhaps unnatural. This can significantly disrupt family relationships, as well as the patient's interaction with friends and professional associates, heightening the sense of isolation and alienation that usually accompanies illness.

The highly technical world of modern medicine usually defines a patient solely in terms of the physical problem, then guides the treatment accordingly, an approach that is often detrimental to physical well-being. By neglecting psychological and social factors unique to the patient, by objectifying that individual, medical personnel disregard information about his or her emotional life that often has a considerable impact on the diagnosis, treatment, and prognosis of the disease.

Feel Good Again explores a fundamental aspect of the universal experience of being sick, which is that all illness simultaneously affects both mind and body. Although a given disease may manifest itself predominantly as physical symptoms (e.g., kidney failure) or mental changes (e.g., schizophrenia), it is actually the constant interaction of a patient's physical makeup, emotional functioning, and social environment that accurately defines the illness. This book explores the implications of that reality for all constituents of the health care system—patient, family, and medical personnel. My hope is that it will give you an appreciation of how medical treatment must focus on the whole person by acknowledging idiosyncratic needs and concerns. That knowledge should help you cope with the stress of illness in your life or the lives of loved ones.

1

Treating Mind and Body

The Biopsychosocial Model

When we compare a bout with the flu to a heart attack or diabetes, it may seem difficult at first thought to establish any similarities. The flu is little more than an annoyance, especially in contrast to the severity and life-threatening nature of heart disease or the chronic conditions accompanying diabetes. Nonetheless, all these illnesses are *identical occurrences*, in the sense that each produces obvious, often predictable, *emotional* changes in the patient.

Any illness, however major or minor, alters the *psychobiologic balance*, the interaction between emotional (psychologic) and physical (biologic) functioning. This interaction is very much a two-way street; just as emotional stress can predispose someone to physical ailments, such as tension headaches, so too can physical illness often cause disruptive emotional responses. During periods of any illness, the body no longer functions in a routine fashion. Although this is most readily perceived in the form of physical symptoms—such as abdominal pain or impaired

5

vision—powerful emotional reactions also accompany illness. Yet these emotional responses are frequently undetected or ignored by patient and physician alike, even though they may have a considerable impact by impeding, even preventing, the recovery from illness.

To provide good medical care, health care workers must have an understanding of what an illness means to a particular patient at a specific time in his or her life, and must tailor the treatment accordingly. They must therefore recognize the psychological and social forces affecting the patient, in addition to understanding the physical ailment. This approach, which requires simultaneous attention to mind and body, is known as the *biopsychosocial* model of medical practice. It regards the patient as a person with unique fears, wishes, and needs. This is in contrast to the cause-and-effect approach taught in medical school, the *biomedical* model, which advocates treating the physical aspects of a disease while ignoring its overall impact on the patient.

As suggested by its name, the biopsychosocial model is a comprehensive treatment approach: the prefix *bio* refers to the biological aspects of a given disease; the term *psycho* refers to relevant emotional issues that disease stirs in a patient; and *social* refers to a myriad of social issues affecting or affected by a particular disease. The biopsychosocial model is a humanistic approach to medical practice that recognizes the inseparable interrelationship between mind and body and incorporates it into treatment.

The severity of an illness usually determines the intensity of the emotional response to it. It is important to realize, however, that there are many exceptions to this generalization and that *illness is a subjective experience*. Each person brings to any experience—including an episode of ill health—a unique psychological and social background composed of diverse factors, such as cultural and religious influences, past medical history, personality type, and age. Together, these factors cause the individual to form an understanding of the illness that is unique, and one that has a definite impact on the physical condition. Two people with identical symptoms and diseases may have dramatically different perceptions of their illness and consequently have totally dissimilar experiences as patients. A relatively benign illness that might be readily managed by one person may have a devastating effect on another, depending on his or her circumstances both past and present.

An emotional response to a physical illness can clearly aggravate symptoms of the physical disease. Excessive anxiety or depression, for example, can provoke a vicious cycle because that emotional instability, originally precipitated by the illness, often aggravates the physical symptoms. Bronchial asthma provides an excellent example of this phenomenon, which is called a *negative feedback reaction.* The onset of an asthma attack heightens the patient's anxiety, which often causes hyperventilation, a type of rapid breathing that actually increases breathing difficulty.

Similarly, a patient's depressed feelings may become so pronounced that he or she may simply give up and become negligent or unconcerned about his or her health. When that happens, the patient often becomes more and more dependent and less likely to assist in his or her own care, and the eventual return to work or social functioning becomes that much more difficult.

Most people have heard about a noncompliant patient, one who may have stopped taking medication or refused an important diagnostic procedure. There are reasons for such seemingly unreasonable behavior during illness. The noncompliant patient is often angered by his or her debilitated, helpless state; unable to discuss feelings, he or she becomes uncooperative.

Feelings such as anxiety, depression, anger, and sadness are all usually experienced to varying degrees and for varying lengths of time by *all* patients. Such emotional responses occur throughout the course of an illness, from its onset through the recuperative phase. They can range in intensity from relatively mild feelings of irritability and helplessness experienced by someone with the flu, to the emotional upheaval caused by terminal illness.

It is an unfortunate reality that emotional responses to

illness frequently go unnoticed or are perceived by patients (and often their physicians) as abnormal occurrences that should be minimized or even ignored. Most people can easily recognize the impact of a disease on their bodies; few are willing or able to recognize its impact on their minds, except in extreme cases of illness or injury, such as residual paralysis following a stroke or the amputation of a limb. The collective pressure to ignore the emotions that accompany physical illness comes from doctors, from family and friends, from the media. Physicians are taught to recognize and treat physical problems and symptoms; family and friends tend to dismiss emotional changes that come with illness as extraneous to being sick. Those patients who are aware of their distressing feelings frequently minimize or deny them, believing it is wrong to exhibit those emotions. The following case study demonstrates the emotional turmoil that can result from such an attitude.

Case Study: Eric Taylor

When brought to the hospital in a coma by his college roommate, twenty-two-year-old Eric Taylor was diagnosed as diabetic and treated acutely. Placed on a regular regimen of insulin and a controlled diet, he was discharged from the hospital within ten days. At that time, he had no noticeable symptoms, and shortly thereafter he returned to his regular classes. During the next two months he felt well physically and his blood sugar level remained in the normal range.

However, during that time Mr. Taylor grew uncharacteristically irritable and more withdrawn than normal. He became increasingly distant from his friends, broke off with his steady girlfriend, and started doing poorly in several courses. During a routine visit to his physician, he reported some of these changes. He attributed them to his diabetes and, despite feeling well physically, complained that he was not receiving the correct treatment. When questioned about this, he also related that he had been sleeping poorly, primarily because of some disturbing dreams in which he saw himself dying under various circumstances: in battle, in a car crash, or as a result of a sports injury. He mentioned that he had found himself crying "for no reason at all" on several occasions and that this had scared him.

When his physician asked why he had not been told about these symptoms, Mr. Taylor was surprised, saying that he did not classify his "outbursts" as symptoms. He admitted being ashamed of his recent behavior and became increasingly determined to hide his supposed weakness from family and friends. He felt that being a diabetic was hard enough—he did not want to be an "emotional basket case" as well. Furthermore, he couldn't understand the drastic changes he had undergone during the past six months. He went from being a personable, gregarious young man, an honor student, and a varsity athlete who was seriously contemplating marriage, to what he described as "a wreck, a nothing." The only way he could explain this change was by blaming his illness, saying "the diabetes is doing this to me," and he angrily demanded that the physician try some other treatment, despite the fact that the results of all his tests were normal. He impulsively decided to stop using insulin because "it wasn't helping anyway," and this resulted in a progressive increase in his blood sugar level, which culminated in readmission to the hospital.

Eric Taylor was correct in attributing his recent behavior to his diabetes. But the change was not due to the physical manifestations of the disease. It was the emotional impact of his illness, his growing comprehension that because of the diabetes he was in some important way "different" from before. It was this self-perception that caused his changed behavior, the sleep disturbance and distressing dreams, the crying episodes, and his diminished concentration on his school work. *He was depressed, and he didn't know it.*

Depression is an extremely common reaction to a diagnosis; yet many doctors and patients are unaware of its existence or its importance as a component of a physical illness. Mr. Taylor attributed the change in his behavior to physical causes. When it was suggested that he was depressed, he agreed, saying, "sure I'm depressed. I don't want to be sick all my life." It was not until that point that he actually acknowledged the emotional impact of his diagnosis. When asked to elaborate on his statement, he became more animated, speaking rapidly and punctuating his speech with frequent jabs of his hand. He wanted to get married, but he was not sure his girlfriend would still want to marry him, and he was afraid to discuss it with her. He wanted to go to graduate school but feared that he would be unable to meet the academic demands. He even wondered if "any school would accept a diabetic." He had considered the idea of trying out for a professional sports team but now felt that he would have to abandon athletics altogether. He felt pitied by his peers, which infuriated him and caused him to drift away from his friends and increasingly into his own private world. He was afraid he would be denied a driver's license because he could "black out at any time." He was also angry at his physicians because they'd "been treating diabetes for so long," and there is still no cure.

Listening to Mr. Taylor, it became increasingly evident why he felt frightened, angry, and depressed about his illness. He had legitimate concerns about his ability to lead the full life that a twenty-two-year-old envisions for himself. However, he also had unrealistic fears about his illness: for example, a diabetic uncle of his had never lost driving privileges despite a stormy thirty-year course with the disease. Mr. Taylor was currently functioning far below his usual level of competence. His social, academic, and athletic skills were certainly impaired at this point; but he was far from the "nothing," the cripple, he perceived himself to be. His entire self-image was distorted, and this impaired his ability to be objective about his illness and interfered with his relationship with his physician, the foundation of any successful medical treatment.

During his rehospitalization the psychiatrist visited Mr. Taylor regularly. Initially they discussed everyday topics such as school and the Boston Red Sox. These conversations helped Mr. Taylor by reminding him that there was a world outside the hospital in which he would have to participate. People with physical illnesses, even those who are hospitalized, still have many of the same concerns about day-to-day living that healthy people have. By not treating Mr. Taylor like an invalid, the therapist was trying to divorce him of the notion that he was in some way crippled and unable to participate in his regular life.

After visiting Mr. Taylor for a few days, the psychiatrist was asked to "give [him] a lecture" on diabetes. His patient was full of questions about the disease, questions reflecting his current fears. During the course of the conversation (which rarely focused on the physical illness), Mr. Taylor began to understand that his recent behavior was an acceptable response to the onset of illness, particularly a chronic illness. His fear about the effects of diabetes on his body, his depression about the course of the disease, his anger with friends who were not afflicted by illness and with physicians who could not restore him to his prediabetic existence—*all these feelings are normal feelings that can surface when an individual becomes ill.* In fact, nearly everyone who becomes ill experiences such feelings. They are usually present to a lesser degree with minor illnesses, but they are still present. The abnormal aspect of Mr. Taylor's response to diabetes was his determined attempt to hide the presence of these feelings from himself and others. Because of his particular predilection for isolating himself from people when under stress, he had no outlet for his growing reservoir of negative feelings. Consequently, they began to overwhelm him. He tried to keep them to himself but communicated them in behavior such as angrily withdrawing from friends, discontinuing his insulin, and demanding alternative treatment from physicians. Only when he began to verbally express and confront his fears, wishes, and needs concerning his illness did he begin to realistically assess the impact of diabetes on his life. As a result, he gradually regained control over his feelings and again felt confident, competent, and strong enough to tackle his illness aggressively, as if he were facing an opponent on the football field.

Eric Taylor's case illustrates how the *biopsychosocial approach* can be used successfully and how important it is to recognize and deal with the emotional aspects of illness. Without proper attention to his emotions, Mr. Taylor would have condemned himself to a difficult and lonely course with his illness. Once he began understanding that he was indeed normal, he became increasingly able to deal with his frustration and sadness in an appropriate way. His clinical depression remitted, and he resumed his insulin therapy.

This chapter has highlighted a universal truth: *emotions affect the response to treatment and thus the course of an illness*. Failure to recognize and deal with that emotional response—whatever form it may take—can, as we have seen, have an extremely detrimental effect.

Even with a long-term or chronic disorder, a healthy emotional attitude makes the course of the disease less difficult for the patient and for family members and friends. To encourage such attitudes, medical care must actively address the mind-body interaction, thereby promoting optimal treatment and preventing unnecessary suffering. This requires that patient and family, as well as physician, fully appreciate what an illness means to the patient at a particular point in time. The patient and physician can then forge a necessary alliance based on mutual understanding and trust, which will encourage and enable recovery in a timely manner.

2

Illness Dynamics

The impact of illness is a unique experience. During every phase of illness a variety of factors converge, causing us to perceive, evaluate, and protect ourselves emotionally against the loss of health in an extremely subjective manner. Pneumonia, for example, is a different experience for a college freshman than for a middle-age widow, even if both patients require the same medications, similar restrictions on activity, and identical measures designed to prevent potential complications. We all have specific strengths and handicaps that characterize our responses to episodes of illness, and which consequently influence the courses of treatment. The interplay between family and cultural background, emotional state, and medical history defines a unique, individual standard by which each of us evaluates and responds to disease. This matrix is our *illness dynamics*, a blueprint by which we—and our physicians—can gain a better understanding of what our personal responses to illness will be.

As illustrated by the biopsychosocial model discussed in Chapter 1, both physical and nonphysical issues are part of the disease process. The nonphysical issues can transform the same ailment into vastly different illnesses for different patients. Everyone lives within a distinctive psychosocial context that may be either beneficial or detrimental when illness strikes. Consider that premise in terms of the following two men who suffered heart attacks with similar damage to the heart muscle. Their histories highlight the many psychosocial factors that influenced when, and to what degree, they became ill, as well as their responses to treatment and their ultimate prognosis.

Case Studies: Albert Lagano and Harold Bushnell

Albert Lagano, a forty-year-old widower, is a mid-level manager diligently working his way up the corporate ladder while supporting two young children. In addition to family responsibilities and professional obligations, he devotes considerable time to a flourishing relationship with a co-worker he hopes to marry. His past history is significant for the unexpected death of his mother from a cerebral stroke when he was thirteen years old.

Harold Bushnell is a sixty-three-year-old executive vice president in a manufacturing firm, on the threshold of retirement. Married to his wife for forty years, he is eagerly anticipating more leisure time with her and his grown children. Mr. Bushnell has consistently enjoyed good health; in fact, his only major medical event, the planned surgical removal of his gallbladder, caused minimal disruption to his life. Although Mr. Bushnell's father died of cancer at the age of seventy, his mother, siblings, wife, and children are all in good health.

After surviving the immediate threat of death, each man manifested a unique reaction to his damaged heart. Mr. Lagano's initial anxiety was progressively superseded by a growing sense of helplessness. The death of his mother while he was so young sensitized him to loss and affected his psychological development by enhancing the normal dependent yearnings everyone feels. Moreover, because she died of cardiovascular illness, he associated his own heart disease with her sudden demise. He also identified with his children's concerns, for he had experienced the same kind of anxiety that comes from recognizing that one's future is largely dependent on the welfare of a single parent. When Mr. Lagano considered the impact of his illness on the course of his career and on the developing relationship with his girlfriend, significant feelings of anger and depression arose. All these factors contributed to a heightened emotional response to his heart attack, which made it more difficult for him to resolve his intense feelings and, in turn, fostered an increased helplessness and dependency on those around him.

Mr. Bushnell was also angered and depressed by his misfortune, cursing the illness that was interfering with the stage of his life he had set aside for relaxation. But the intensity of his feelings was tempered by the knowledge that his family was grown and could take care of themselves, that his spouse had consistently provided reassurance and support when needed, that he had already realized his professional ambitions, and that he was financially secure. For these reasons, Harold Bushnell was more easily able to work through the emotions provoked by his physical impairment and quickly returned to his previous level of functioning.

Albert Lagano and Harold Bushnell each suffered the same degree of heart damage, but each reacted to the period of ill health in a different fashion owing to the impact of distinctive psychological and social factors.

The relationship between biologic status, emotional makeup, and the supports and stresses of the social milieu constitutes a person's individual illness dynamics. This idiosyncratic standard, which represents the understanding of a specific disease during a particular time in life, is portrayed schematically in Figure 1. The shaded area defines the illness dynamics: the distinctive interrelationship between the conscious and unconscious psychosocial fac-

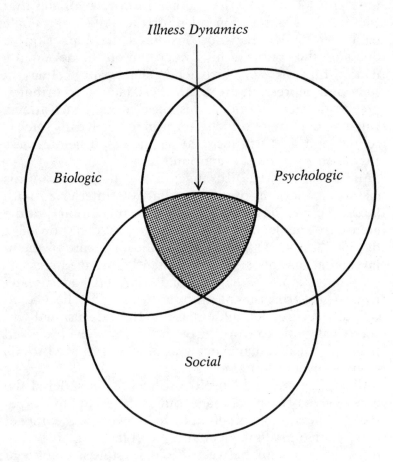

Illness Dynamics

Biologic

Psychologic

Social

Figure 1

tors affecting and affected by biologic status. Illness dynamics incline the individual to assess any and all information related to the illness in light of personal values, wishes, needs, and fears; they are what determine the manner of responding to the illness. Because there are always different factors interacting, each person reacts to illness subjectively, influenced by the unique components of his or her illness dynamics.

Illness dynamics can, and do, predispose us to certain diseases and protect us against others. For example, if diabetes is prevalent in a woman's family, a *biologic* component of her illness dynamics increases the risk of developing the disease because of its hereditary nature, whereas a *psychologic* component heightens concern about that possibility. She may be predisposed to increased anxiety if routine blood tests reveal a high normal blood sugar level, even though her general health is good. Similarly, most patients would be better able to cope with an episode of ill health if the social aspect of their illness dynamics included strong supports, like an extended, caring family. In this manner, the illness dynamics provide a "map" that patient and physician can use as a blueprint to assess or even predict the response to an illness at a given time in life.

Both Mr. Lagano and Mr. Bushnell shared the common life-threatening experience of a heart attack, but their illness dynamics were very dissimilar. The most significant biological component of Mr. Lagano's illness dynamics was his mother's genetic endowment. Mr. Lagano's excessive dependency was an important psychologic component of his illness response. Also contributing to his significant depression was his stage in the life cycle, since the heart attack occurred at a time when most individuals are focused on the challenges and joys of life, rather than on the fear of death. In the social sphere, Mr. Lagano's heart disease had a considerable effect on the two young children whose welfare depended on his wage-earning ability. This lack of flexibility within the family system placed even greater stress on him to recuperate rapidly and completely. In contrast, consider Mr. Bushnell's life: his physical resilience, psychological strength, and the supports of his social network combined to help him readily negotiate this difficult period of ill health.

Figure 2 illustrates the distinctive illness dynamics of these two men. The diagram shows how psychological and social issues transformed a heart attack into vastly different illness experiences for Mr. Lagano and Mr. Bushnell. By programming a few factors into the three areas that determine illness dynamics, we get an immediate biopsychosocial picture of these two men that is quite distinctive.

Consider, then, the uniqueness of any patient's illness dynamics, given the myriad of possible psychological, social, and biological issues at work. Individuals with the exact same disease can react completely differently with their families and physicians because of the individual factors that make up their illness dynamics.

Biologic Components of Illness Dynamics

Within the sphere of biologic components, the specific illness in question is perhaps the most important factor. Generally speaking, the more benign and self-limited the disease, the more readily we can grieve the loss of health and move on with life. With a less serious illness, we are more likely to recognize that the condition will have only a minimum effect on overall functioning. On the other hand, catastrophic illness is more likely to produce an abnormal response, because acceptance of permanent debility is a considerable emotional task for anyone. The issue of short-term illness versus a chronic, long-term disorder will also have an impact on our reaction. Some people handle an acute disease process better than others, knowing that while matters may be serious at the moment, they will not be ill forever. Others adjust better to chronic illness: the familiarity of symptoms, no matter how uncomfortable, may be peculiarly reassuring. Such individ-

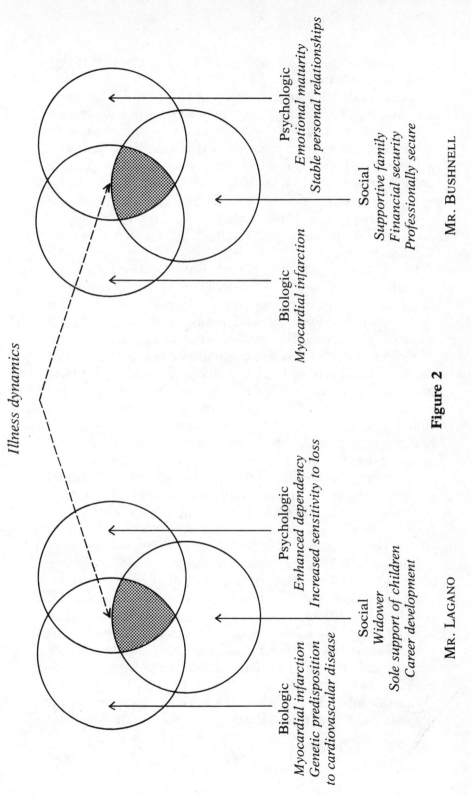

Illness dynamics

Psychologic
Emotional maturity
Stable personal relationships

Social
Supportive family
Financial security
Professionally secure

Biologic
Myocardial infarction

Mr. Bushnell

Psychologic
Enhanced dependency
Increased sensitivity to loss

Social
Widower
Sole support of children
Career development

Biologic
Myocardial infarction
Genetic predisposition
to cardiovascular disease

Mr. Lagano

Figure 2

uals experience the sudden onset of sickness as terribly anxiety provoking.

Individuals vary greatly in their vulnerability to physical illness. The reasons for this variation range from simple factors, such as age, to progressively more complex issues, such as allergic reactions to necessary medications. An abscessed tooth, for example, may represent only a painful annoyance to a healthy young adult, or a potential source of serious infection to a diabetic, or a grave threat to a cancer patient whose ability to fight infection may be seriously compromised by many of the medications used for chemotherapy.

Previous episodes of ill health produce a selective vulnerability to subsequent illness. Prior abdominal surgery places a person at greater risk for intestinal obstruction as a result of adhesions, and major surgical procedures increase the probability of common postoperative complications. Most people are quite aware of their particular constitutional strengths and vulnerabilities. Attempts to measure such vulnerabilities may be extremely objective or strikingly unrealistic, with consequent effects on the illness response.

Biologic heritage can also have a considerable effect on illness dynamics. Someone who is "genetically loaded" for a particular disease frequently has a heightened emotional response when suggestive signs and symptoms appear. Patti Beaumont was hospitalized for a brain abscess resulting from a bacterial infection of a bone in her foot. Although thoroughly knowledgeable about her medical condition, she became preoccupied with the idea that her abscess marked the onset of Huntington's Chorea, the neurological disorder that caused her father's death. Ms. Beaumont was completely aware of the details surrounding her case and was given considerable reassurance that she was not suffering from Huntington's Chorea. Nonetheless, the abscess and the involvement of her brain provoked unpleasant associations.

Considerable denial is another way in which some people respond to their hereditary predisposition. Brian Powers, a middle-age man whose entire family succumbed to heart disease, denied obvious symptoms of a heart attack before seeking emergency medical attention. Prior to this episode, he had lived a type-A life-style—a competitive, aggressive, hard-driving existence, dictated by endless responsibilities and deadlines—unconcerned that his behavior might activate a presumed predisposition to heart disease. No physician can predict how a person will interpret his or her medical heritage when becoming ill, but providing the doctor with the information needed—both objective facts and subjective feelings—helps facilitate treatment of both body and mind.

Obviously, the specifics of the particular illness can have significant psychological and social effects. Iris Terrell, age twenty-seven, needs a hysterectomy for cancer of the cervix. Because she is young, and childless, she may have a difficult time adjusting to both her illness and the necessary treatment. Certain kinds of illness, particularly those affecting the central nervous system, can interfere with the ability to come to terms with poor health. The delirium produced by meningitis or the aphasia (the loss or impairment of speech) resulting from a stroke can prevent a realistic assessment of the impact of illness on daily life, let alone a resolution of the varied emotions connected with such a plight. Whether an illness is congenital or acquired must also be considered. The ramifications of being born deaf are far different from the ramifications of losing the sense of hearing after already knowing how to speak.

Finally, the pharmacologic treatment of disease can be an important component of the illness dynamics. Most patients do respond therapeutically to medications, though many drugs have numerous side effects ranging from an upset stomach to impotence to mental confusion. Drugs may also cause distinctly adverse reactions, including allergic responses that may be relatively mild or have a serious impact on various organ systems. Certain medications, such as narcotics and tranquilizers, have an addictive potential. In addition to providing relief for symptoms, medications can cause discomfort, alter mood, or place some patients in potential danger. For all these reasons, pharmacotherapy may play a significant role in shaping the individual illness dynamics.

Psychological Components of Illness Dynamics

One of the most significant determinants of a person's illness dynamics, in both a positive and a negative way, is his or her personality. In the most general terms, personality refers to an individual's predictable response pattern to stimuli. From the external environment or internal thoughts that spontaneously spring to mind, whether pleasurable or unpleasant, any stimulus will trigger characteristic patterns of behavior that constitute a particular personality or character style. Generally speaking, these patterned responses become much more pronounced when a person must contend with strong, diverse emotions such as those precipitated by illness. Someone who is normally somewhat obsessional tends to become even more rigidly controlled in the face of illness; a person who is excessively dramatic might become even more attention-seeking. Reversion to familiar patterns has been shown to be an adaptive response to stress, but in the extreme this can also evolve into self-defeating conduct.

At the age of fifty-seven, Samuel Floyd was diagnosed as having a hernia that required surgery. Mr. Floyd's personality can be described as somewhat obsessive: he is rigid in his beliefs and often disguises his true emotions. These personality traits, which became amplified after Mr. Floyd's diagnosis, interfered in his relationship with his physician. Doubts about the appropriateness and effectiveness of his treatment prompted an endless series of questions, observations, even complaints, concerning the surgery and follow-up care. Whereas increased communication between patient and doctor almost always facilitates medical care, Mr. Floyd's behavior, a reflection of the obsessive anxiety characteristic of his particular personality, had the opposite effect. He became increasingly irritating to his doctor, which hindered the development of a collaborative relationship between them. Similarly, dependent individuals, those who characteristically abdicate responsibility for their welfare to others, have considerable difficulty attaining an emotional perspective on illness.

Overall psychological health, closely linked to personality type, is an important component of one's illness dynamics. In general, the greater a person's psychological health, the greater the ability to assess the impact of illness accurately. Mature psychological coping mechanisms, such as anticipation, humor, and sublimation, facilitate a productive, helpful emotional reaction to illness. An individual who relies heavily on unhealthy mechanisms such as denial, distortion, and projection is obviously handicapped in this regard. Such patients define their own reality by opting to see only what they want, particularly when stressed. Under such circumstances, it would be impossible to acknowledge accurately and gain perspective on the feelings accompanying an episode of illness.

At each age, different psychological stages have a bearing on the illness dynamics. Adolescents, for example, generally feel omnipotent. This predisposes teenagers toward denial of illness. An unfortunate consequence of this denial is noncompliance with required medical treatment, such as the dietary indiscretions or inconsistent use of insulin often found among juvenile diabetics. The geriatric patient, already faced with accelerated physical decline, is often quite despairing about the additional burdens brought on by sickness. This can complicate overall care, by predisposing elderly patients to excessive anxiety or depression when they become sick. It may also interfere with a necessary adaptive aspect of aging, namely, coming to terms with one's mortality. This normal process can become pathologic if the usual concerns about dying are transformed into morbid preoccupations with a prolonged, uncomfortable death due to the onset of significant illness late in life.

Previous encounters with sickness can affect the illness dynamics surrounding subsequent instances of ill health. John Baker, age thirty-five, had an episode of prostatitis. The pain of this flare-up unexpectedly forced him to curtail his sexual activity. Any suggestive urinary symptoms occurring at a later date, even if they are unrelated, could provoke strong feelings associated with memories of the prostatitis. In addition, unanticipated complications as a result of medical care, such as postoperative pneumonia or an allergic reaction to radiologic dye, can affect future reactions to illness. The onset of any symptom can provoke unpleasant memories of previous treatment and cause anxiety, anger, or depression. Or any new abnormality might be denied in an attempt to avoid being a patient once again, a condition subconsciously associated with discomfort and a threat to well-being.

Even when the physician is unaware of the specific determinants of a person's illness dynamics, his or her medical history may provide a reasonably accurate prediction of the reaction to current ill health. When Howard Barbour told his physician that he had been hospitalized for three weeks for an uncomplicated appendectomy, an extremely long period for that medical condition, his doctor realized that Mr. Barbour might characteristically become excessively dependent when ill. Mr. Barbour, for example, might have delayed or avoided early discharge from the hospital, possibly by exaggerating his discomfort from minor symptoms, because he preferred the supportive hospital environment to the responsibilities that awaited him at home. Realizing that this problem might recur during Mr. Barbour's admission for another, unrelated condition, his physician took steps to avert the problem, by emphasizing the anticipated length of hospitalization and arranging for additional support during the early convalescent period at home.

People who develop diagnosable mental disorders in response to major life crises, such as divorce or termination from a job, are at greater risk of responding to medical illness in a similar fashion and may experience a recurrence of their psychiatric illness. They can become clini- cally depressed, suffer from pathologic anxiety, relapse into alcohol or drug abuse, or even lose touch with reality through a recurring psychotic illness such as schizophre- nia. Mood swings, the cyclic fluctuations of emotions be- tween mania (euphoric highs) and depression (oppressive lows), also affect the illness dynamics. Someone who is manic, and feels consumed by feelings of happiness and well-being, may discount or even fail to recognize obvious physical symptoms. That person is more likely to shrug off the concerns expressed by family members and dismiss the physician's advice. Depression, on the other hand, often diminishes a patient's motivation to get well. Phys- ical illness can also aggravate certain psychiatric illnesses. For example, individuals who have diminished mental functioning due to dementia often become increasingly confused, disoriented, and have greater loss of memory when subjected to additional physical stress. The varied effects of an illness, including infection, an elevated tem- perature causing mild dehydration, or even the effects of general anesthesia, can all have this impact.

Social Components of Illness Dynamics

If close relationships are based on a healthy interdepen- dence characterized by shared responsibilities and mutual support, life's varied stresses, including illness, can be ac- commodated. However, some relationships are more rigid, with strictly defined roles being maintained to preserve a marriage or family unit; in these cases, illness can have an extensive—and sometimes devastating—effect.

Donald Chase worked as a loan officer in a savings bank. His wife, Sally, stayed at home with their two children, and he maintained the role of primary wage earner. When he developed a back problem that required surgery and was hospitalized and bedridden for a number of months, Mr. Chase was forced into a new role: that of the dependent spouse. Because so much of his self-esteem was related to his role as wage earner, and because the dynamics of his family were centered on him in that role, he became quite depressed. Other people in a similar situation might become resentful or experience some other discomfort; these feelings are often mirrored by family members who must also assume different positions of responsibility. The new balance in a relationship between patient and family may be contentious and negative, detrimental to someone attempting to recognize and resolve all the emotions associated with illness.

Similarly, major illness in a child can place great demands on the parents' time, energy, and finances, sometimes becoming an all-consuming preoccupation that stresses every area of the family's existence. Many compromises and material sacrifices must be made. Nevertheless, an understanding, supportive family can help the child come to grips with and accommodate to his or her disease. A less empathic family can actually compound the difficulties brought on by sickness, thereby decreasing the chances of the child adjusting emotionally to the stress. This is also true in the case of a sick, elderly relative or spouse whose declining years are marred by lengthy illness.

Position in a nuclear family can also affect the illness dynamics. It is true that some lifelong patterns prevail as a consequence of birth order. Older siblings tend to be more autonomous, and younger ones tend to be more dependent, characteristics that can become even more conspicuous during periods of stress. During his hospitalization, a man who was the tenth child of fifteen had to wait while a definitive diagnostic procedure was postponed four times, an occurrence that would infuriate most patients, but which failed to anger him. When asked how he maintained his composure, he stated that his early years had taught him to "wait his turn." His philosophic reply was quite understandable given his family background and the persistence of childhood patterns.

Interpersonal functioning—educational and occupational experiences, as well as the status of personal friendships or marriage—can have a bearing on illness dynamics. For example, a highly ambitious and competitive middle-aged executive could suffer a great deal of psychological conflict in the aftermath of a major heart attack. In addition to dealing with the difficult task of accepting the diminished autonomy brought on by his disease, he would also have to cope with the possible loss of income and authority.

Apart from any genetic predisposition to disease passed on through generations of ancestors, we also inherit systems of beliefs concerning illness and illness behavior from our families. Someone who witnessed a parent's long struggle with a chronic disease can easily regard all illness in a pessimistic light. Consciously or unconsciously, illness represents to that person an existence marked by repeated contacts with physicians, frequent hospital stays, and physical decline despite numerous prescriptions, medications, and treatment regimens. In short, sickness becomes synonymous with suffering, invalidism, death, and all the emotional pain surrounding it. Raised in that kind of environment, this individual may be seriously handicapped in any efforts to make a positive accommodation to illness.

Similarly, the attitudes toward sickness that prevailed in the family during childhood can greatly influence one's illness dynamics throughout life. In some families, the presence of any symptom—minor or major—is good cause to call the doctor. Although these families make a considerable investment in terms of time, energy, and money, they feel the price is worth the reassurances of good health. Children raised in this kind of family can become conditioned to this illness behavior and may maintain it throughout their lives. On the other hand, there are many families that are intolerant of sickness, viewing it more as a stigma than as something that requires medical attention. Denial of illness then becomes an institutionalized norm within the family, and violation of that norm invites criticism or abuse—powerful incentives to suffer stoically and silently.

Harry Conover, a young farmer from West Virginia, was brought to the Emergency Room disoriented and in a semi-coma. Upon examination, it was discovered that he suffered from a serious, previously undiagnosed abnormality of his kidneys, resulting from a birth defect. When Harry's parents were contacted, they acknowledged that their son had been generally less vigorous and productive than his siblings, but they minimized the importance of this behavior because "he kept on working." The family's standards for illness were abnormally stringent, but they were never questioned by Harry, who maintained the same unrealistic stoical behavior. The myth of a family's invincibility owing to generations of superb health, folk remedies, and holistic cures can have detrimental effects on any individual who is attempting a reasonable accommodation to the impact of illness.

Cultural background can also have considerable bearing on one's illness dynamics. Researchers have found characteristic patterns of thinking and behavior concerning various aspects of diagnosis and treatment within specific ethnic groups. Some become exceedingly emotional, if not overly dramatic, when confronted with illness, whereas others remain stoically accepting or overly concerned with the *facts* of illness as opposed to the *emotions* it produces. Medical personnel may be unaware of the effects of long-standing, broad-based social values on the perception of illness. Educating them about a patient's ethnic heritage can help them understand how this cultural group normally responds to illness and thus shed light on the patient's response. They are then alerted to detrimental health behaviors, such as the denial of significant symptoms, which the patient might consider to be normal.

Each of us has a specific and unique set of illness dynamics composed of a multitude of factors. Some people readily reveal many of these factors to health care providers during the course of their treatment; others may offer only a superficial view of the biologic, emotional, and social forces that shape their particular illness response. In such cases, more responsibility is placed on the caretaker to elicit those necessary responses.

In order to obtain comprehensive medical care, two things must occur. First, the physician or other health care provider has to take a detailed history—one that includes not only the facts and the details of the medical care but also the pertinent social and psychological details. This most certainly involves a degree of probing and insightful questioning. Second, the patient and family must discover what the illness dynamics are and how they are affecting the situation. (This will also enhance the quality of the history the physician documents.) For the patient, this self-knowledge is crucial; it can both empower him or her and restore the feeling of being in control. This confidence is essential to coping with the sometimes frightening, often confusing and dehumanizing, medical system.

3

Grieving the Loss of Health

We all experience the pain of loss at some time in our lives, resulting from a variety of circumstances. The loss of a loved one or the loss of self-esteem that results from such disappointments as professional setbacks or a rejection in love are universal experiences. Although each of these events is distinctive, with unique implications for different individuals, they do have something in common: the emotional experience they provoke in us. *The psychological response to a loss is shared by all.* Psychiatrists call the normal response to loss a *grief reaction*, a time-limited period of mourning, usually lasting six weeks to six months, during which we accommodate to the loss. Grieving allows a comprehension of our loss on both an emotional and an intellectual level. This is necessary in order for us to adjust to the changes caused by the event and then get on with life.

The grief reaction is a process. It occurs in stages, with predictable emotional (and often physiological) changes at each stage. Experiencing the different stages of grief and incorporating these new understandings into daily

life—the process of mourning—is important in and of itself. If the process didn't occur, we would be in the position
of trying to "turn off" emotions, an unhealthy situation
with an impossible goal since feelings are bound to
emerge, either directly or indirectly. Initiating the grief
process is the all-important first step toward accepting the
loss.

At the end of the grieving period, feelings stabilize. Although coping with day-to-day responsibilities may not
always be done as effectively as before the loss occurred,
we now return to more normal functioning. The level of
that functioning, however, is largely dependent on the particular loss that has been suffered. This final reequilibra-
tion, the resolution of all feelings, is necessary in order to
come to terms effectively with the particular loss.

Typical Grief

The grief process is well-illustrated by the occurrence of
a death in the family. The first stage of grieving is *denial,*
a reaction of shocked disbelief—"But I just saw him last
Sunday!" or "Doctor, are you sure that she has really
died?" Some people react to the news with shock and are
seemingly incapable of responding. This stage is generally
brief, usually lasting only a few hours, although some form
of denial often persists for several days; for example, a
woman believes she sees her dead husband walking down
the street. When all manifestations of denial are gone, and
the loss is experienced as completely real, there is a progression to the next stage, which is characterized by feelings of *anger.*

Although longer than the period of denial, the anger
stage is also relatively short, lasting from several days to
several weeks. At this point, the full intensity and range
of feelings become more apparent. People at this stage
commonly experience some or all of the following emotions: irritability, resentfulness, argumentativeness, and
possibly even rage. All these feelings, which may be gen-

eralized or directed specifically at someone, are completely normal. They are symbolic of our natural attempt to make sense out of death, to find someone or something to blame for our anguish. When something bad happens, when people suffer, it is natural to try to search for a reasonable and acceptable explanation. Bereaved people may direct angry feelings toward the physician for presumed negligence or insensitivity to the needs of the deceased. Someone may feel angry with himself or herself, self-critical of real or imagined failure to be sufficiently loving and supportive to the deceased during his or her life or period of illness. Hostility is also commonly felt toward the dead person, fostered by a feeling of having been abandoned by the loved one, obliged to carry on alone.

As the initial emotional turmoil begins to wane, an increased sensitivity to the loss develops. At this point, a sadness evolves, characterizing the *depression* phase of the grief reaction. This stage, with its pronounced emotional and physical components, is what usually comes to mind when we remember a period of grieving. A pervasive sadness and feelings of emptiness, isolation, despair, and helplessness commonly arise. Bereavement often brings withdrawal from the social milieu or professional responsibilities, owing to lack of interest in anything but family matters. A preoccupation with memories of the deceased develops, and considerable time is spent reminiscing.

Obvious physical changes accompany this phase of grief, including sleep disturbances (such as insomnia or early awakening); appetite disturbances (such as anorexia or excessive eating); lethargy; fatigue; inability to concentrate; memory loss or forgetfulness; and decreased sexual interest. Existing physical illnesses may become aggravated—an ulcer might flare up or chest pain from angina may occur more frequently. New symptoms—often vague aches and pains—may develop. The depression stage, more than any other phase of the grief reaction, is a time when the bereaved person is most clearly self-absorbed.

This normal stage in a grief reaction closely resembles

a clinical depression, a psychiatric disorder characterized by specific, objective symptoms (see Chapter 8). Symptoms during the depression phase of a grief reaction are usually less intense than the more debilitating symptoms of a clinical depression. Moreover, normal grief is self-limiting, whereas depression requires treatment in the form of psychotherapy, psychoactive medications, or a combination of both.

Many people at this stage of a normal grief reaction worry that there might be "something wrong" with them. The person suffering from this kind of distress may genuinely appear to be seriously depressed and worried that he or she is suffering from some kind of a major psychiatric illness. This is not usually the case. Time and emotional energy are most focused on the loss, and this inward focusing ultimately leads to the development of a new psychological equilibrium that allows the person to continue life without the love and support of the deceased. With time, the bereaved usually becomes increasingly accepting of the loss and eventually returns to normal functioning. The role of other family members and friends at this time is extremely important. They can help reassure the bereaved that feelings of sadness and depression are part of normal grief and will remit with time.

The grieving process reaches a conclusion in the *acceptance* or *resolution* stage. At this point, intense feelings—both positive and negative—about the deceased progressively diminish, and they begin to be placed in some kind of perspective. Normal grieving must involve remembering both the "good" and the "bad" about the person and confronting all feelings. Only then is it possible to come to some kind of closure, or resolution, which enables the bereaved to live with the pain of the loss. While it would be neither desirable nor possible to simply forget the person who has died, the one left behind must eventually come to the realization that life has to continue despite this tragic loss. Although this may sound harsh, it is the only option if he or she is to pick up the pieces and continue living a normal life.

As this emotional readjustment occurs, changes in behavior begin to reflect increased acceptance of the loss. The progressive emergence from the protective cocoon spun during the mourning period permits a renewed interest in life. In general, the individual becomes more outwardly directed. The details of everyday life become more routine, more normal. Simultaneously, physiologic functioning returns to its previous state, as symptoms that characterized the depression disappear.

The process of grieving is a comprehensive psychologic and physiologic response that enables us to comprehend a loss emotionally as well as intellectually. We readjust to a world that is missing someone very dear to us. This process of reequilibrating is normal; it is not merely anticipated, it is required. Failure to adapt to losses in this manner is restricting and may even be harmful. Indeed, some individuals are so totally unable to accept such losses that they retreat into a world of despair and themselves die shortly after their beloved.

Normal grief, then, gives us the opportunity to examine and place into perspective a wide range of feelings following a painful loss. By going through the process of grieving, we allow ourselves to feel *all* our emotions in an appropriate manner. This enables us to get on with the business of living without being stressed by an excessive or debilitating emotional burden.

Grieving the Loss of Health

The death of a loved one is an obvious and most painful loss, but we regularly suffer other significant losses that have considerable impact on our emotional lives. The loss of health caused by physical illness is one such occurrence. Like the death of a loved one, it precipitates a grief reaction. Ill health is usually defined by the patient in terms of *concrete*, obvious manifestations of a pronounced illness that causes permanent physical changes. Blindness or the amputation of a limb is an easily recognizable physical deficit requiring a person to acknowledge the *literal loss of health* in a functional or anatomic sense because of new restrictions on independence. However, even a minor illness—one causing no lasting changes in physical state—can precipitate feelings of loss. That is because sickness has a *symbolic*, as well as a real, significance for everyone. Once the real *and* the symbolic impact of a physical ailment are understood, the person can begin to comprehend the important connection between an illness and the process of normal grief.

There are several reasons for the symbolism inherent in an episode of illness. Taken in its most general sense, sickness, particularly a major or chronic case, forces us to accept that we are not immortal. The fantasy of being forever well and living indefinitely is a holdover from childhood, when we behaved as if we were all-powerful and indestructible. But sometimes illness does not cause us to doubt our omnipotence, as illustrated by the heart attack patient who refuses to follow his diet, or continues to smoke, believing that "nothing bad can really happen to me."

The realization that we are not immortal is a simple but staggering truth. It usually occurs when we confront illness in either ourselves, a family member, or a close associate. *That realization causes us to suffer a tremendous loss*, in some ways a loss of innocence. After having weathered the flu or a fractured wrist, we feel more vulnerable. While a certain amount of vulnerability is desirable so that we may confront reality and take any necessary action when we are ill, too much vulnerability can make us feel less in control of our life than we previously were. These are not usually persistent, conscious feelings that affect day-to-day life. Such concerns are instead incorporated into our consciousness as we mature, and our recognition of them is clearly enhanced by an episode of illness.

Case Study: Martha Thomas

Martha Thomas suffered a ruptured disc in her back three years ago. She did not require surgery but did spend many weeks in traction. After she had been pain free for six months, her physician allowed her to resume all her activities. But Ms. Thomas is still afraid to swim, something she formerly enjoyed. What causes Ms. Thomas's seemingly irrational fear? No doubt she has some conscious concern that excessive strain could cause recurrence of disc symptoms. More important, though, are the unconscious memories related to her injury. Many emotional cues regarding that event—the frustration of being confined to bed, her self-directed anger for possibly causing the injury, her fear of another bout with prolonged pain—can remain outside of conscious awareness. Even after the specific details of the situation are long forgotten, the emotions connected to them are retained in Ms. Thomas's unconscious and influence her day-to-day behavior.

Psychiatrists call this phenomenon *repression*, which may be defined as "selective forgetting." Certain thoughts and feelings in deep recesses of the mind can exert an unrecognized influence on individuals, particularly during periods of stress, such as prolonged illness. The individual who has difficulty accepting the return to health, like Ms. Thomas, or the person unable to grieve the loss of health, must identify and understand certain repressed thoughts in order to overcome those situations.

In addition to undermining the feeling of omnipotence, illness conveys *specific* symbolic meanings to individuals because of their distinctive illness dynamics. These messages can interfere with the ability to grieve the loss of health. Consider the following two cases of middle-age men who experienced the same degree of loss of health. Robert Anderson, an active, competitive man, suffered a mild heart attack at the age of forty-two. He recovered physically; however, since his father died at the age of fifty as a result of a stroke, he has retained an obsessive fear of any symptoms suggesting continued abnormalities of his cardiovascular system. For example, he took his own pulse up to ten times every hour, becoming quite anxious if it exceeded a certain rate. Consequently, even though he has recovered physically, his long-standing fear of heart disease, caused by memories of his father's death, has significantly impeded his emotional recovery and interfered with his social, occupational, and recreational life.

Philip Darrow, age sixty-five, also suffered a heart attack. However, because both of his parents died of gastrointestinal disease, he more readily accepted the onset of cardiovascular disease as a fact of later life, aided by the knowledge that his illness had no serious aftereffects. If, on the other hand, he were to develop an ulcer, it might greatly distress him because of his association with his parents' fatal illnesses.

Whether impaired health is experienced in the literal sense, as a result of clear limitations in physical functioning, or in the abstract symbolic sense, the same psychological response is *always* present. In every case *illness* is accompanied by a natural grieving process during which the patient mourns the previous state of health. This process is analogous to the grief reaction caused by the death of a loved one. Illness forces the patient to confront and acknowledge a new level of physical functioning. Only after working through all the strong feelings about this altered physical functioning can the patient fully accept these deficits and proceed with life. Acceptance helps reestablish an emotional equilibrium and facilitates lifestyle changes that may be necessary in order to live with the particular illness.

Working through feelings about the loss of health is a multistep process. First, the patient must identify all the feelings the illness or disability has aroused, realizing that they comprise a wide *variety of emotions*. Next, he or she must understand where all those feelings come from, in order to gain some perspective on the extent of each emotion. This ultimately allows the patient to arrive at an acceptance of the illness, which makes grieving the loss of health an adaptive process.

Just as incomplete grieving following the death of a loved one can progress to emotional, and even physical, illness, nonacceptance of the loss of health can have similarly detrimental effects. There are individuals suffering from heart disease or from ulcers who are unable to acknowledge their true state of health. They commit dietary indiscretions that result in bouts of congestive heart failure or abdominal pain. These people actually aggravate their medical problems through their inability to put into perspective all the feelings precipitated by the illness. Consequently, the feelings emerge in other ways and prohibit resumption of a normal, productive life. The emotional acceptance of an illness or disability is a crucial phase in physical recovery. Acceptance does not mean liking the illness. In fact, to effectively cope with illness, it is just as important to acknowledge and understand what is disliked about the illness, and how that makes the patient feel.

A medical or surgical patient may frequently feel "out of control" during various phases of an illness—from its acute onset, through the period of convalescence, even over the years of its chronic course. Such helplessness is caused by the recognition of one's own mortality, as well as by the fact that the body may not be performing as desired. For these reasons, the patient frequently is out of control. Chapters 10 and 11 detail measures that can be taken to regain control.

The first step in regaining control is to acknowledge the loss, proceed through the normal stages of grief, and ultimately make some kind of peace with this new, different physical condition. Once this acceptance is achieved, it is possible to deal more knowledgeably and productively with medical caregivers and maximize the potential to continue living a happy, productive life. Family or other members of the patient's support system, too, by going through the grief process, will be able to increase their understanding of the illness and in that way assist the patient in taking charge of his or her medical care.

Case Study: Gary Laughlin

Gary Laughlin, a fifty-year-old nurse, has been afflicted with persistent kidney infections for more than a decade. The kidneys serve an important role in regulating the blood pressure; because of the extent of renal damage caused by his repeated infections, Mr. Laughlin is now suffering the consequences of uncontrolled hypertension. The first acutely life-threatening consequence of his illness—a heart attack five or six years ago—unleashed the stages of the grief process.

Mr. Laughlin was at work in the hospital when he developed a pain he attributed to indigestion. When the pain increased, he was examined by a staff doctor who diagnosed chest inflammation and sent him home. The next day, however, Mr. Laughlin's pain worsened, and he called the doctor, who told him he was being neurotic.

A couple of weeks later the pain returned. Mr. Laughlin consulted another doctor, who did an electrocardiogram and made arrangements for hospitalization the next day. Mr. Laughlin, who didn't want to wake the doctor, endured a night of severe pain before he finally called him early the next morning and went to the hospital.

Mr. Laughlin had arrhythmias (irregular heartbeats) and was in the intensive care unit for seven days. He spent another three weeks in a ward and an additional month recuperating at home. While hospitalized, he was anxious about the time he was losing from a new job, feeling quite helpless and depressed.

This case history clearly illustrates the different stages of the grief reaction as a result of illness, starting with Mr. Laughlin's initial denial and culminating in his approach toward acceptance.

The first stage of the grief reaction is denial, and Mr. Laughlin's initial denial was pronounced. As a nurse, he was trained to recognize the signs and symptoms of medical problems. Yet when he developed chest pain, he accepted a diagnosis of chest inflammation even though he knew that heart disease is a common consequence of hypertension and that a major symptom of a heart attack is chest pain. When the pain intensified, he accepted a doctor's insensitive—and inaccurate—assessment that he was being neurotic, even though he had never dramatized or exaggerated any medical problems before. Finally, when his condition deteriorated to the point where he was having severe pain during the night before a scheduled admission to the hospital, he delayed calling his doctor.

What causes a person who is suffering from severe pain—in this case, a person who should have known better—to act in a seemingly irrational manner? Mr. Laughlin's behavior reflected his wish to ignore or minimize the signs that he was seriously ill. Denial regularly permits us to adjust to stressful situations by protecting us from unpleasant feelings that might otherwise overwhelm us. However, it becomes counterproductive, even dangerous, when we try to discount obvious, severe pain in an effort to minimize our emotions.

When denial breaks down, feelings of *anger* begin to surface. Anger permits the focusing of feelings in order to begin to try to make sense out of the irrational. Mr. Laughlin's anger was evident; he spoke loudly, in clipped, curt sentences, and was somewhat challenging. He talked of his several physicians and how none of them had cured him; he wondered if they had treated him incorrectly and criticized them for not providing him with a true and accurate assessment of his condition over the years. He was angry with his current physician, who had not yet been able to control effectively Laughlin's rising blood pressure, and whose unavailability kept his patient uninformed about various test results.

Gary Laughlin was most explicit in describing the *depressed* phase of his grieving process. He thought that he was "pretty young" to have a heart attack and was worried about his work. Would he be able to keep his job during a lengthy recuperation? Would he be physically able to handle it, or any other job, in the future? Forced at an early age to confront the loss of health, Mr. Laughlin's feelings were completely normal. But there was something

else involved aside from these anticipated concerns, something that added tremendously to the overall stress Mr.
Laughlin's heart attack caused. Here was an active, independent individual who was confined to bed. Rather
than feeling autonomous as he was used to, Mr. Laughlin
felt helpless and, in his words, "terribly depressed." The
feeling was compounded by the fact that he was knowledgeable about medicine but could actively do nothing to
improve his health. He had to rest passively in bed and
place himself completely in the hands of his doctors and
fate. Unaccustomed to inactivity, and to feeling out of control, he was depressed.

To regain control of his life and get back to his old
self, Mr. Laughlin had to move beyond depression and
come to some acceptance of his illness. As he conva-
lesced at home, his depression began to diminish. When
he described his return to work, he became considerably brighter and more animated. He had survived a life-
threatening illness, acknowledged his fears and concerns,
and succeeded in putting those feelings behind him. Neither his physical nor his emotional state prevented him
from resuming his previous activities and active control
of his professional life.

In reviewing this case history, we see that Mr. Laughlin's
feelings included denial of obvious symptoms of a heart
attack; anger at his physicians for never adequately controlling his blood pressure; depression caused by his
enforced inactivity while hospitalized; and finally, acceptance of his illness, allowing him to continue functioning
effectively despite his chronic illness. With the passage of
time, he was able to put these feelings into perspective
and eventually integrate them into his life. By acknowledging his physical limitations but not allowing them to
ruin his outlook, Gary Laughlin had empowered himself
to go on living a happy, productive life, in spite of severe,
chronic illness.

If someone is unable to adapt emotionally to a physical
illness, unresolved feelings can become an emotional bur-

den with long-reaching, even fatal effects on health. An inappropriate or incomplete grief reaction to an illness can either directly interfere with specific medical treatment or indirectly lead to general neglect of physical well-being. In either case, daily functioning, as well as family life, social relationships, and work, can be adversely affected.

When a person is unable to come to terms with the realities of a changed physical condition, he or she becomes mired in one of the phases of the grief process and preoccupied with the feelings characteristic of that stage. That emotion is then expressed toward family and friends and affects these relationships. The impact is usually negative, given the emotions of grief. People who get stuck in the anger phase, for example, tend to alienate friends, loved ones, and caretakers. As a result of their bitterness, people in this stage tend to irritate the very people they depend on for support and care. Patients who act depressed, overly anxious, or helplessly dependent tend to be extremely demanding of those around them, with similarly negative effects. And people who get stuck in the denial stage tend to frustrate family members, friends, and caretakers, all of whom are aware of realities that the patient refuses to acknowledge.

In such maladaptive responses to illness, the sick person cannot come to terms with physical illness because he or she is so preoccupied with the negative feelings precipitated by his or her loss. This sets up a vicious cycle. When people close to the patient react to this negative behavior, it further alienates the patient, and the maladaptive cycle continues, often endangering important relationships and sometimes causing a permanent rupture. A period of mourning is a time for reflection and thought: by its very nature, it is a lonely time. Alienating the affections of the people who care most when their support is needed most is self-destructive and dangerous.

Case Study: Emily Barnum

Emily Barnum is seventy-one years old and has an eleven-year history of high blood pressure, which has progressively weakened her heart. Her physician asked a therapist to visit her in the hospital, where she had been admitted for congestive heart failure, a condition characterized by the accumulation of excess fluid in the body due to the heart's weakened state. The doctor was puzzled by her present status; a relatively mild cardiac impairment did not adequately explain her recent deterioration. Ms. Barnum and the therapist met for the first time in her hospital room. As part of the usual history taking, she was asked about prior hospitalizations. At that time, she revealed the most significant aspect of her medical history: the amputation of her leg in 1971. That episode affected all of her subsequent health care, including the current illness and hospitalization.

The therapist asked Ms. Barnum about the amputation. She said it had been necessary because of a blood clot in one of the arteries in her leg. She did not know how she got the clot and claimed the news that she would require an amputation came as a complete surprise. She believed she had let the doctors know there was something wrong with her leg. She regretted that she did not protest loudly enough about the leg while, in her view, the doctors were preoccupied with her heart and blood pressure.

In fact, Ms. Barnum's doctors were well aware of her high blood pressure, congestive heart failure, and vascular obstruction of her leg, but were much more successful in treating the former. Despite the fact that her leg problem was less debilitating than her heart disease, it was a chronic condition that progressed steadily despite vigorous and appropriate treatment. She had been informed of the possibility of amputation; nevertheless, Ms. Barnum blamed the clinic for what she perceived as bad medical treatment.

During the next part of her talk with the therapist, Ms. Barnum detailed the limitations of her current life, attributing them to her disease. She enumerated a number of complaints that were clearly symptoms of clinical depression. She reported a lack of appetite over the past four years and an inability to fall asleep. She said that whenever she couldn't fall asleep, she would think about her leg and fear that she had become a burden to family and friends. Ms. Barnum also said that she didn't express her feelings of helplessness to anybody, not even her husband, and that she held back many other things as well. She felt ill-fated but preferred not to say so and didn't know why.

Ms. Barnum related how her life had gone downhill after her surgery. She severely limited all housework, abandoned her hobby of quilting, and stopped traveling. She also gave up driving. Most important, she completely discontinued her daily routine of visiting neighborhood friends. Her social contacts became limited to friends calling on her, and over the years these visits became increasingly infrequent. Physical changes accompanied her self-imposed limitations: her diminished appetite resulted in progressive weight loss, and her inability to fall asleep at night, accompanied by ruminations about her amputation, contributed to her chronic fatigue.

Emily Barnum did not realize that the changes in her level of functioning and capacity to enjoy life were not solely the result of her physical handicap. She also suffered from her obvious difficulty in resolving the powerful and painful emotions unleashed when her leg was amputated. These emotions were quite apparent during the session with the therapist. Although she tried to minimize it, her anger at her physicians was blatant. She portrayed them as ignorant, insensitive, neglectful, and condescending, and claimed they ignored her complaints about leg pain because she "did not holler loud enough." She suppressed her resentment, even from her husband, and the consequences of her silence were tragic. Her unexpressed anger festered, daily strengthening her conviction that she was a victim, and she lived her life accordingly. She gradually withdrew from the world. Emily Barnum was on a sitdown strike, and her suffering was largely self-imposed.

After the meeting, the therapist wondered if Ms. Barnum's resentment of physicians had reached the point where she was angrily—and covertly—rejecting their current treatment. She had mentioned that her low-salt diet and cardiac medications were not necessary "all the time," even though she'd been clearly and repeatedly told that they were. The therapist suspected that her recent hospitalizations were necessitated by her deliberate inattention to a prescribed medical regime, a self-destructive acting out of her anger. Had she directly expressed those feelings from the outset, especially to her physicians, she would have been able to minimize the emotional pain that now complicated her treatment.

The inability to grieve effectively the losses suffered as a result of illness causes an abnormal psychological reaction to that illness. Emily Barnum is a striking example of this phenomenon. Her pervasive, but muted, anger fostered her social isolation, depression, and probable noncompliance with her medical treatment. In effect, she was ruining her life. That is a staggering price to pay for being unable to deal effectively with the angry feelings unleashed by her illness.

The inability to grieve the loss of health results in an abnormal psychological reaction to illness. These reactions usually take the form of excessive denial, anger, and depression, though anxiety and pronounced dependency are also common. Anxiety is often a variant of anger; some people ventilate hostility by feeling excessively anxious. Dependency is a reflection of depression, a *behavioral* expression of the helplessness experienced by the depressed individual. Each of these emotional conditions occurs during the normal grief response, but in that condition the individual ultimately resolves these conflicting feelings. In an abnormal illness response, however, he or she becomes preoccupied with one of these emotions and persists in reacting to the illness solely from that emotion's perspective. Alternatively, the person might completely deny the presence of any feelings accompanying the loss of health.

4

Coping with Illness

Coping and Crisis

When something upsets our biological and psychological equilibrium, our usual behaviors come into play to help overcome the particular stress and reestablish a balance. This is accomplished through such personal problem-solving mechanisms as talking about concerns with relatives and friends, asking for advice and support, or planning necessary life changes to accommodate to the situation. This process enables us to manage or *cope* with stresses—including the stress of illness—without an overwhelming and permanent sense of disruption or loss of control.

Sometimes, however, stress causes such a degree of turmoil that our usual mechanisms are inadequate to handle the problem. In these times of *crisis*, our thinking becomes less rational, and the accompanying intense emotions we experience—such as anger, anxiety, depression, guilt, and fear—can cause even more disorganization of thought.

All crises are self-limited; they will come to some kind of resolution within a given time frame. How beneficial

46

that end result will be depends on the actions taken by the person (or people) in crisis. Coping, then, involves the resolution of a crisis in order to relieve turmoil and disorganization. But there are actually two types of coping—*adaptive* and *maladaptive*. In a healthy adaptation, the ultimate result is the definitive resolution of a particular stressful situation, as well as personal growth and maturation. By attaining mastery over a situation and being as active as possible in its resolution, we are better able to put it into a realistic perspective and move on with life. A maladaptive response, on the other hand, often produces psychological regression. When this happens, we use less effective patterns for dealing with emotional difficulties. The crisis will eventually resolve; however, we will have less control over how that happens, because we have passively allowed events to unfold. We are less in control of the actual circumstances of life and, consequently, less in control of emotional life.

There are two basic components to coping, an *emotional* and a *cognitive* process. In the former, we gain mastery over our emotions by working through those feelings via grieving, as discussed in the preceding chapter. Adaptive coping also involves a cognitive process, during which we obtain specific information about a given stress. That knowledge helps us manage some of the emotions unleashed by the crisis. For example, learning that severe abdominal pain is due to appendicitis, a readily treatable ailment, alleviates anxiety that symptoms might be due to a fatal illness. Knowledge also helps us recognize the specifics of what needs to be done to help resolve a crisis.

Coping, then, is an emotional and problem-solving activity for meeting life's stresses. By applying emotional and cognitive resources to deal with these challenges, we can successfully resolve the specific crisis and reestablish as much autonomous functioning as possible depending on the severity of the particular stress. Adaptive coping has an impact on relationships (for example, returning to the usual family patterns that existed before a member suffered a life-threatening heart attack); on physical activity (for example, regaining as much function as is possible following a stroke); and on emotional functioning (for example, not being overly depressed or anxious while convalescing from surgery).

Tasks for Coping with Illness

Rudolf Moos, a researcher concerned with various behaviors during illness, discusses specific tasks that must be accomplished in order to cope adaptively with the impact of physical illness. Some of these tasks are uniquely concerned with the disease; others are general issues relating to the state of being in crisis. Issues that fall into the first group include: dealing with physical limitations and pain; dealing with the environment of the medical world; and learning how to work collaboratively with health care providers. Issues that fall into the second group include: preserving a sense of emotional balance; maintaining a satisfactory self-image; preserving important relationships; and preparing for the uncertainties that the illness can bring.

A fundamental task for adaptively coping with illness involves *dealing with physical limitations (such as blindness, the inability to walk, or even a restricted diet), as well as pain and discomfort,* which may be caused by the disease and/or medical treatment. Zbigniew Lipowski, a psychiatrist long interested in the relationship between physical symptoms and emotional behavior, describes *tackling*, one response that helps patients accomplish these goals. *Tackling* means actively taking on the challenges and hardships of an illness—such as prolonged, often difficult physical rehabilitation after a stroke. This counteracts physical symptoms and fosters a feeling of mastery over the situation. Tackling usually involves setting particular goals regarding the illness and actively pursuing them. When a man who is recovering from back surgery promises himself he will be playing tennis by a certain date, he is practicing this coping style. He pushes himself to get out of his hospital bed, to do prescribed exercises regularly, and to increase his level of activity incrementally in order to get well as quickly as possible. This approach is diametrically opposed to that of patients who simply choose not to deal with their limitations, in a kind of "out of sight, out of mind" mentality. Although such denial may reduce the stress of the illness, it is maladaptive coping, because these individuals are subject to negative and restrictive circumstances.

Another adaptive coping task specifically related to disease involves *dealing with the workings of the medical world*, an environment foreign to most people until illness strikes them or someone close to them. A variety of circumstances provoke strong emotional reactions in patients and their families, such as meeting with unknown specialists; undergoing sophisticated diagnostic tests; being hospitalized and caught up in a strange daily routine; receiving special treatments such as chemotherapy, physical rehabilitation, and speech therapy; and dealing with unpleasant consequences or limited progress of those treatments (see Chapter 11).

Learning how to be open and trusting with health care providers requires the abdication of a measure of autonomy to unknown caregivers. Patients must develop relationships with new doctors and other personnel (such as nurses, specialized therapists, dieticians) who have a considerable effect on the overall experience of hospitalization. The same applies to personnel who work in the offices of doctors that patients must visit for follow-up care.

The same general coping tasks that help a person deal successfully with any other life crisis come into play when contending with an episode of illness. It's important to work hard to *preserve a sense of emotional balance* so as not to become overwhelmed by intense feelings. The grieving process creates powerful emotions, and patients must reassure themselves that they will not lose control of these emotions. One coping behavior that helps accomplish this task is *minimization*. People often minimize the facts of an issue in order to prevent an initial emotional overreaction.

By thinking of a breast lump as a lump, and not immediately equating it with cancer, a woman helps limit the degree of her anxiety, which might otherwise become debilitating. Another coping mechanism is called *vigilant focusing*. This involves taking an extremely intellectualized approach to the illness. By "not seeing the forest for the trees," some patients avoid the overwhelming feelings caused by the stress of illness until they are better able to put the episode into a broader perspective. For example, in the initial period following a heart attack, a patient's concern about heart-rate regularity helps control strong emotions about the long-term effects of heart disease. Another adaptive coping behavior is called *reasoned learning* about the illness. Becoming knowledgeable about congenital causes of an illness may help alleviate guilt and self-directed anger about having contributed to, or created, one's own health problems. Alternatively, learning how certain behaviors may have endangered one's health may motivate an individual toward more beneficial actions, such as dietary changes designed to lower an elevated serum cholesterol level. Reasoned learning also relates to treatment, such as becoming knowledgeable about medications and their side effects, the importance of specialized diets, and the details of specialized treatments such as dialysis. Finally, the patient may try to find a meaning to, or reason for, the illness. This philosophical approach, a very human exercise, is often useful in helping to maintain an emotional balance.

It is essential to *maintain a satisfactory self-image*. In the face of a disease that brings both real and symbolic losses, the patient must try to remember that a person is never exclusively defined in terms of health or illness. It is especially important to recognize and review personal strengths, to have self-confidence. The patient must remember that he or she is liked and respected by friends, and loved and cared for by family. It is important for the patient to remain involved in family matters. Even during a hospitalization, it's possible, for example, to keep abreast of childrens' school performances, their extracurricular activities, and social lives. If confined, in traction, to a hospital bed for weeks, professional contacts should be maintained, wherever possible, to help keep the mind occupied while the body is healing.

The patient must also work at *preserving interpersonal relationships*. This may be difficult during a hospitalization, because the usual opportunities for communication are disrupted. But having an illness should not mean that a person must abandon the people in his or her life and become increasingly withdrawn and self-absorbed. The patient must actively fight off isolation in order to prevent its progression into alienation. This keeps the patient connected to his or her social world and also elicits needed support from loved ones and friends. Another means of accomplishing this task is to get reassurance through feedback from others knowledgeable about a particular health problem. All patients want to know whether their feelings and moods are "normal." Two good sources of this information are health care personnel and others with the same or a similar kind of illness. Self-help support groups exist in many communities, hospitals, and even physicians' offices, for such diverse health problems as diabetes, heart disease, seizure disorders, and AIDS. Many people are greatly reassured by learning that what they're experiencing is not uncommon; it helps them cope.

It is important to *prepare for the uncertainties that the illness might bring*. Although no one can know the future, it is possible to look at the potential difficulties that might develop and prepare contingency plans. Martin O'Donnell, a forty-seven-year-old who was an avid jogger, suffered a serious knee injury that required him to stop exercising. Martin had to think about what his injury meant: would he have to turn to another form of recreation and exercise, such as swimming, that would put less strain on his weak knee? By *anticipating* the possibilities for the future— imagining a range of possible, as well as improbable, scenarios—Mr. O'Donnell was able to prepare himself for some of the feelings he would probably experience during the course of his illness. This intellectual assessment of the potential outcomes of an illness often provides a preview of the various emotions that accompany those outcomes. In this manner the patient's feelings become less intense and thus less likely to prove overwhelming during the course of an illness.

Individual Coping Strategies

Individuals have varying abilities to accomplish the several tasks involved in coping adaptively with an episode of illness. Individual illness dynamics determine which tasks are easily achieved, which ones are difficult, and which are impossible. Alfred Thompson, for example, has a long history of heart disease and diabetes, and has been hospitalized six times over the last six years. His most recent stay lasted close to two months. Mr. Thompson is obviously familiar with hospital routine and has even developed ongoing relationships with many of the personnel during his several stays. Consequently, he is able to adjust quite easily to being hospitalized and can even get some reassurance from the routine. Knowledge about how to use a hospitalization to his advantage has helped Mr. Thompson's recovery during several critical periods. On the other hand, for someone who is a loner, interested mainly in solitary pursuits, the task of establishing productive relationships with medical personnel, and of preserving relationships with family and friends, can be extremely difficult during hospitalization.

This relationship between illness dynamics and the ease or difficulty of accomplishing specific tasks of adaptive coping determines what type of *coping strategies* are employed by patients. Based on a study of how individuals combine different types of coping behaviors, Lipowski has identified different types of *coping strategies*, which may be adaptive or maladaptive to a particular patient.

The first strategy views *illness as a challenge,* where the patient strives to "beat" his or her sickness and regain control. This obviously adaptive response to illness benefits the patient, as well as everyone close to him or her.

Some people view their *illness as an enemy,* an invader that needs to be repelled. This type of thinking is more common in the case of an infectious disease, where patients can think of antibiotics as "wiping out" the invading germs, or in cancer, where patients often visualize their chemotherapy as bullets or weapons that attack the tumor. This coping strategy may involve more imagined than real control over an illness. However, it still provides patients with a positive sense of mastery that, even in the short run, helps their adaptive coping.

Viewing an *illness as punishment* is not uncommon. Some patients passively accept being sick and do little to improve their physical or emotional well-being. A long-term smoker suffering from emphysema may merely accept his or her symptoms as the consequences of a self-destructive habit—and even continue smoking. This coping strategy is obviously maladaptive; the individual resolves the crisis by basically giving up.

Some patients view *illness as a weakness,* equating their ill health with a failing of some kind, even if it is due to chance (such as a congenital abnormality, a hereditary disease, or even an auto accident). An adaptive way of dealing with this view would be to equate recovery with not being weak. The patient would try to demonstrate regained strength by overcoming the illness. But if the patient views illness as confirmation of the fact that he or she is *meant* to be weak, that person is more likely to passively accept fate and not work through the feelings associated with the illness by grieving the loss of health.

There are people who actually welcome being sick, viewing *illness as a relief* from the responsibilities of work, family, or financial obligations. People who resolve the crisis of illness in this manner may actually be more secure and emotionally calm when they are ill. This coping strategy is also characteristic of individuals who are hypochondriacal, many of whom invoke their complaints and imagined illnesses to absolve themselves from life's day-to-day demands.

Finally, there are some people who respond to *illness (even a minor one) as an overhwelming, irredeemable loss.* Bettina Jackson, age thirty-one, is the kind of person who places great emphasis on her physical appearance. She is always well-dressed and watches her weight. When injuries from a car accident caused a scar on her forehead, she was devastated. Unfortunately for Ms. Jackson, the only way she could resolve the psychic turmoil caused by the (minor) alteration in her appearance was to completely retreat from her previous routines and relationships. Her entire life-style changed: she remained indoors and rarely saw people. Although the disorder in her life caused by the crisis of illness was resolved, it was at a tremendous price.

Just as illness dynamics cause the individual to perceive illness in a unique fashion, which greatly influences the ability to grieve the loss of health, so too do they affect the ability to manage the crisis of illness, by shaping coping strategies that may be adaptive or nonadaptive. Adaptive coping strategies can help patients deal with the stress of illness by maximizing control over the situation; whereas those that are nonadaptive can actually perpetuate the illness state. Both adaptive and nonadaptive coping behaviors help resolve the turmoil and the intense emotions accompanying the crisis of illness. However, only the former allow patients to accept the losses incurred by ill health and maintain as much autonomous functioning and as high a quality of life as is possible, given the circumstances of their particular health problem.

How Families Cope

Coping with illness is very much a family affair. The lives of family members, and often close friends, are greatly affected when a loved one becomes ill. Family members go through the same cognitive and emotional changes that the patient experiences, and the family, as a unit, often resorts to a characteristic coping strategy. In general, the healthier the family prior to the illness of one of its members, the easier it will be for the family to cope with that particular stress. Characteristics that reflect the psychological health of a family include cohesiveness of the family unit, an ease and ability to express feelings among members, a low level of conflict within the family, and independence of the individual family members. Conversely, the more pathologic the family prior to the stress of illness in a member—the greater the degree of anger or helplessness or anxiety that characterizes usual interaction—the poorer the family will cope with the stress.

Families also have to perform certain tasks during the coping process. These family tasks, like those of the patient, either are related directly to the illness or are more general in nature. The family must first learn about the illness—the short-term and permanent impairments that can accompany an illness; what type of rehabilitation is useful or necessary; prognosis; and potential complications. More general coping tasks include dealing with the patient's emotions and their own feelings about the situation, as well as establishing new types of interactions and relationships within the family (either long-term or for the duration of the acute phase) when they are required by the circumstances of the patient's illness.

These tasks vary during the different phases of a patient's clinical course, and correspond to the family's staged response to an illness, which is detailed in Chapter 10. For example, a heart attack victim's family can speak at great length to the doctors, who can outline the different stages of this life-threatening event. The doctors can explain the treatment regimen at each phase and discuss what the long-term effects are likely to be. By gathering information, a cognitive aspect of coping, the family can mobilize into action at a time when they are still numbed by the acute impact of the illness. This helps them make specific, potentially lifesaving decisions (such as whether to allow the patient to be resuscitated if he or she suffers cardiac arrest) and generally helps them feel more in control of the situation.

After the initial phase of an illness, families frequently

experience a tremendous outpouring of feelings from which they had previously been distracted by the requirements of critical decision making. Once that happens, families must cope with these emotions and their impact on the patients.

Depending on the circumstances of illness, a family may have to tend to tasks that are more cognitive, or more emotional, or more related to the social relationships or the financial issues of the patient and family. The impact of the specific illness on the particular patient, combined with the impact of the patient's illness on the particular family, will shape the family's coping process; hence each family's experience is unique.

Some families, like some individuals, can perform certain coping tasks but not others. Families that are emotionally constricted, for example, may have an easier time dealing cognitively with an illness. They may better handle the acute or rehabilitative stage, while gathering information on the specific goals of physical therapy or chemotherapy and focusing less on their feelings. Families that lack the intellectual skills for understanding the patient's illness often abdicate decision-making responsibilities to the doctors. This can be a double-edged sword, either reassuring the family or making them feel even more out of control. A family like this may have another adaptive coping behavior, however; they may be more open, more expressive of feelings, which facilitates coping by permitting discussion of painful feelings about changes in their lives brought on by a member's illness.

What Makes a Family Able to Cope Adaptively?

If a family is well equipped to cope with the stress of illness, it generally has the ability to shift easily from one type of coping behavior to another. For example, in the case of a chronic problem like Hodgkin's disease, the family may have to adapt frequently to different aspects of the illness—depending on which symptoms predominate during a single episode—or its response to treatment. At one point, the family may have to decide on a particular type of treatment for a specific symptom, requiring them to operate in a more cognitive mode, gathering information and studying the recommendations made by medical personnel. At another point, possibly during a remission, they may be more focused on attaining an emotional equilibrium that comes to grips with the fact that the patient still has a life-threatening illness. The family also needs to be aware that at any time they must be prepared to spring into action and actively involve themselves in responding to an acute flare-up of the illness. A family in this situation is well served by a capacity to employ different coping skills. If they lack that flexibility—or if they are psychologically unhealthy, as characterized by rigidity, authoritarianism, emotional immaturity, or repression—they are more likely to have some unhealthy or pathological resolution of the crisis caused by illness in one of its members.

Case Studies: The Trogi and Coombs Families

The Trogi family is not an emotional family. In fact, they tend to repress or deny their feelings, remaining cold and distant from one another and the people in their lives, because acknowledgment of their feelings is too painful and threatening. As a result, they usually resort to the fight-flight mode of interaction, a distinctly unhealthy behavior pattern. However, the family deals extremely well with the intellectual decisions they must make. Consequently, when Dan Trogi, age fifty-five, had a heart attack, the family was able to get him to the hospital quickly and calmly, to ask appropriate questions about his treatment, and to help him adhere to the necessary treatment regimen during the early weeks of recuperation. However, throughout this period no one in the family ever discussed how they felt about the changes in Mr. Trogi's life and the resulting changes in their own lives. Instead, the feelings emerged insidiously, and growing resentments among family members were acted out. For example, the family began treating Mr. Trogi as an invalid, despite his ability to lead a normal life, thinking they would thereby insure against a relapse and, consequently, another disruption in their own lives. Mr. Trogi responded to this treatment by planning a premature return to work, causing the family to act even more controlling of his activities.

The Coombs family is quite different from the Trogis. John Coombs also had a heart attack, but the degree of the family's emotional involvement in his illness was so great that they lost perspective on his ability to deal with illness. As a result, their lives became increasingly controlled by Mr. Coombs, as they began to neglect important aspects of their own lives. Friendships and social relationships were abandoned because family members preferred to "stay home with Dad." The oldest daughter dropped out of graduate school so she could help out at home and "spend time" with her ailing father. Wendy Coombs became so preoccupied with her husband's illness that she was warned about her declining performance at work. Ironically, individual family members were unable to give Mr. Coombs the kind of emotional support he required, because they were too self-absorbed in their own distress. Both the Trogi and Coombs families had great difficulty coping with illness adaptively, primarily because of their inability to utilize a variety of coping behaviors. As a result, the lives of all the family members were seriously disrupted, while the patients failed to get the emotional support that could have helped them cope with their illnesses.

Some Final Words About Coping

In addition to the illness dynamics, there are general characteristics that can be used to predict how well or poorly individuals will cope when stressed. People whose coping skills are more adaptive are generally more optimistic, predictably looking on the brighter side of a situation. For example, a person who has suffered a heart attack and has started a physical rehabilitation program talks about how much more fit he or she now is as a result. This type of person, rather than viewing the training solely as a way to treat the physical impairment, is able to identify wider-reaching benefits of the exercise program. Good copers are usually more flexible, with the ability to reinterpret a negative situation. They are information seekers who gather facts, learn about their options, and, consequently, are better equipped to determine an adaptation to stressful situations. Good copers, though aware of their emotions, are rarely overwhelmed by those feelings. Such individuals may feel sad, but they will not become so depressed that it interferes with their lives. These individuals are able to recognize and express their feelings, while retaining an appropriate perspective, thereby retaining control over their emotions.

People whose coping is generally nonadaptive also display characteristic behaviors. They often employ excessive denial, not only of emotions, but also of the realities of a particular situation. People who exhibit excessive denial usually have extremely rigid personalities, another characteristic of poor copers. They have a mindset about what they expect to feel and how they "should" act, making it very difficult for them to adapt to new, especially stressful, situations. This behavior makes adaptive problem solving an impossibility.

An alternate consequence of rigidity is passivity, which greatly undermines adaptive coping. Some overly rigid people often do *nothing* when their usual routine fails them and they become ill; it is their only other means of coping. Passivity may paradoxically give way to impulsiveness in some individuals who decide to "just try something" when the usual means of coping fail. The willingness to try anything different often reflects excessive denial, borne of the notion that the individual in question is unable to accurately acknowledge and assess his or her emotions. Many people who seek esoteric cures are at this stage; rather than grieving their actual loss of health, they try to correct the situation with irrational behavior.

Individuals with poor emotional control generally cope

poorly with stress. This is particularly true when they have to deal with intense emotions, such as those that arise during the grief process. These people frequently allow their feelings to build up until they "explode" when greatly stressed. Another characteristic behavior is a tendency to wallow in their emotions, indulging themselves by concentrating on how depressed or helpless they are. Rational decision making, a necessary component for adaptive coping, then becomes difficult, if not impossible.

Coping is both an emotional and a cognitive response that permits mastery over stressful situations. When we are able to cope with a situation, we can adjust to the stress in a way that permits us to return to a baseline level of functioning, or as close to that baseline as is possible given the particular stress. In the case of illness, a major component of coping involves grieving. Patients must acknowledge both the real and imagined losses incurred because of illness by gaining a perspective on all the emotions that are precipitated by it. This kind of self-exploration helps to regulate emotional distress. The cognitive aspect of coping utilizes rational problem solving. In the case of illness, this usually entails making decisions about different aspects of treatment and rehabilitation. The two components of coping help patients resolve their diverse feelings concerning the loss of health, thereby preventing the onset of one of the abnormal responses to illness.

5

The Denial Response

One way of dealing with unpleasantness in our lives is to deny its existence, refusing to accept or even acknowledge disagreeable feelings or thoughts. As an unconscious mechanism, *denial* permits us to ignore certain events and emotions without any awareness of doing so. Unlike other ways of dealing with negative emotions, denial is absolute; that is, it does not modify distressing thoughts or feelings—it negates them.

The child's attempt to deal with worldly fears is a good illustration of how denial works. While visiting the zoo, Billy, an excited six-year-old, repeatedly says "I'm not scared" while staring at the caged lions stalking back and forth—and he is genuinely unafraid. The little girl standing next to him may openly express fear through words or tears, but Billy remains unshaken. By unconsciously exercising denial, he can enjoy the adventure of observing enormous, otherwise terrifying beasts while simultaneously preventing any frightening thoughts from intruding on his pleasure.

Everyone utilizes denial. It permits adjustment to

stressful situations by negating the unpleasant impact of distressing thoughts or extremes of emotions such as excessive anxiety, anger, or depression. Even if we sense that we might be denying something, we still benefit because the potentially detrimental feelings remain outside our consciousness. For example, a woman may feel "unnaturally" calm before an important interview, but experience the full effect of her very real anxiety after the ordeal of the interview is concluded.

We exercise denial to cope with the normal stresses of life. A common example of *adaptive* denial involves the operation of a car. The dangers of driving are obvious and well publicized: tens of thousands of Americans die in traffic accidents annually, and many more are injured. If the average driver were constantly to be aware of these statistics, he or she would never get into the car. However, most of us are not inhibited by such fear. Either we never think about being involved in a car accident, or we dismiss the possibility by reassuring ourselves of our cautiousness and driving skills. Of course, we also try to control our fears by taking sensible precautions, such as using seat belts and driving at a safe speed. Nonetheless, most of the anxiety is automatically defused, placed safely outside consciousness by the adaptive exercise of denial.

Denial is also used to cope with the more global stresses of our lives. Nuclear weaponry, for example, is frequently discussed as an option in military conflict. Nevertheless, national polls demonstrate that the majority of Americans doubt that nuclear war will occur, primarily because it is unthinkable. Inherent in this belief is a great deal of adaptive denial.

Without the ability to deny powerful thoughts and emotions deriving from hundreds of day-to-day situations, we would be incapable of leading normal lives. However, when denial becomes too *defensive*, it becomes maladaptive and detrimental, preventing us from accepting and assessing the realities of life. Examples of this behavior include taking an examination without studying and driving while impaired or disoriented by alcohol. Depending on the situation, the consequences of denial can be grave.

Medical illness is a common stressor to which people frequently react with excessive denial. The fact of being sick, possibly seriously ill, is too frightening for many people; as a result, their reaction to illness can become a nonresponse. Powerful feelings often accompany illness. Fear of being overwhelmed by those emotions causes some people simply to deny the reality of ill health.

Almost everybody knows someone with very real symptoms—possibly suggestive of a critical illness—who ignored or downplayed them until coerced into seeking medical attention. A common example of this response is the middle-age man who, after experiencing chest pain for several days, is finally cajoled by his family into going to the hospital. Despite at least a passing knowledge of the common cardiac symptoms, this patient dismisses questions about his reluctance to seek medical help by calmly reporting to his physician, "I thought it was indigestion." Another example is the elderly woman with slurred speech and mild paralysis on one side of her body who doesn't consider the possibility of a stroke, but instead blames her symptoms on fatigue. These common examples do not represent the normal denial that is the first step of the grieving process (see Chapter 3). They illustrate instead denial that is *excessively defensive,* reflecting patients' ongoing difficulty in accepting the realities implied by their acute symptoms.

People like this deny their illness in a variety of ways. *Displacing* attention onto another part of the body is one such technique. Monica Rinehart, for example, was quite knowledgeable about multiple sclerosis because her mother had died of the disease. Yet when Ms. Rinehart experienced her first episode of optic neuritis, an inflammation of the optic nerve that is a common symptom of the disease, she sought evaluation instead for an oddly shaped wine-colored birthmark, which had never previously concerned her.

Some patients *rationalize* their feelings in an attempt to

deny their concerns. When Harriet Buckman, a heavy smoker, began to feel ill and lose weight, she claimed that she was glad. Instead of voicing concern about the possibility of lung cancer, she told family members that she "needed to lose a few pounds." Other people interrupt their medical evaluations by refusing diagnostic procedures or even leaving the hospital against medical advice. They convince themselves that such decisions are correct without recognizing their true motivations: to deny the reality of illness by making it impossible to collect the necessary medical data.

Excessive denial does protect a person from bearing the painful emotions associated with illness, but it is at the price of placing the patient in peril. Such denial usually dissipates as symptoms of disease intensify—and, it is hoped, before the illness becomes life threatening.

Nevertheless, denial is not necessarily confined to the early stage of illness but can be present during any phase of the disease process. It can occur even before someone becomes sick, as in neglecting such long-term preventive measures as immunizations. It may be present during the early stages of illness, during the acute course (even if hospitalization is required), and into convalescence and aftercare. Denial is even seen in dying patients who adamantly declare their good health in response to attempts by family and friends to say a final good-bye. In all these circumstances, denial is invoked as a defense against the reality of illness—which *does not* have to be terminal, debilitating, or even serious—by those who cannot grieve the loss of health.

Why does one individual utilize denial while another becomes excessively angry and a third becomes helpless and depressed as a means of dealing with illness? At what point during the course of illness does someone invoke denial? Does excessive denial persist indefinitely, or does it eventually give way to a realistic appreciation of the impact of illness? The answers to these questions are determined by an individual's illness dynamics (see Chapter 2), as illustrated by the following cases.

Case Study: Jeffrey Waldman

Twenty-one-year-old Jeffrey Waldman suffers from kidney failure, the result of a bacterial kidney infection he acquired at age five. He was hospitalized for his worsening symptoms: debilitating fatigue, headaches, and dizziness. His symptoms required a new medical regimen with drastic implications for his daily functioning and long-term well-being. Despite a long-standing awareness of his condition, he showed considerable denial about his medical status, his treatment plan, and his view of the future.

Mr. Waldman exhibited a tentative bravado. He admitted he'd had a kidney disease since the age of five but claimed that the doctors never did pinpoint his illness. In fact, he had *repeatedly* been informed of his diagnosis, for he frequently told his physician that he had forgotten "just what's wrong with my kidneys."

A more serious manifestation of Mr. Waldman's denial concerned his attitude toward his treatment regimen. Overexerting himself physically by playing a lot of tennis and disregarding warnings about the dangers of certain foods were part of Mr. Waldman's unconscious attempt to convince himself of his good health. But he paid a heavy price for these actions.

Mr. Waldman recounted his medical history in an indifferent, if not dispassionate manner. He repeatedly attempted to negate the seriousness of his current symptoms by proclaiming his health had been "pretty good" since age five and that "since then nothing has really happened." As evidence of this, he cited his level of activity, his physical conditioning, and his unrestricted diet. Furthermore, he tried to minimize significant symptoms by attributing them to a cold, despite the fact that he had been placed on a variety of medications to lower his blood pressure in an attempt to control his headaches and fatigue. He tolerated his uncomfortable, distressing symptoms until he became too dizzy to function at work; only then did he contact his physician. He was hospitalized at once and placed on dialysis. Mr. Waldman professed surprise at this change in his treatment; but he was, in fact, well aware that dialysis was not only a possibility but a probable next therapeutic step. He attempted to deny this reality by accepting it as a possibility only of later life, yet he had never been given that kind of time frame for his anticipated kidney failure. In fact, the doctor had always been pessimistic about Jeff's prognosis, an opinion she'd voiced to the patient and his family.

Of all the factors responsible for Mr. Waldman's denial response, two in particular stand out: the nature of this illness and his stage in the life cycle. Progressive kidney failure can remain a hidden process for many years. Although Mr. Waldman intellectually understood the implications of his ailment, he denied his emotional response until his symptoms actively interfered with his functioning. An aggravating condition was the fact that the progression of his illness occurred during adolescence, normally a time when one struggles to carve out an independent identity and become increasingly free from parental control. This developmental stage is usually accompanied by an enhanced sense of omnipotence. Dependency needs are often hidden behind a facade characterized by contempt and disregard for any support or guidance by elders. Medical illness can make the adolescent passage even more treacherous by posing an additional threat to emerging independence and, consequently, provoking an even more extreme stance of omnipotence. This can result in a frightening neglect of medical realities, which in Mr. Waldman's case contributed to a behavior that was detrimental to his health.

Because denial had interfered with his ability to grieve effectively for the loss of his kidneys, Jeff Waldman failed to seek treatment until he suffered an obvious, physical decline—excessive fatigue and crippling headaches. This denial prevented him from pursuing treatment to inhibit the progression of his disease. Fortunately, Mr. Waldman's denial never reached life-threatening proportions. Despite his active life-style, his weakened condition ultimately obliged him to acknowledge his physical decline.

Case Study: Thomas Hall

The case of Thomas Hall illustrates denial during the acute phase of a disease process. Mr. Hall, a forty-six-year-old architect, has phlebitis of one leg complicated by pulmonary emboli, blood clots that break off from the inflamed vein and eventually lodge in the lungs. With correct treatment, the illness usually clears; however, it is potentially fatal if neglected. Mr. Hall denied the significance of alarming signs and painful symptoms, despite being aware of both their presence and their implications.

Mr. Hall said that he was admitted to the hospital for severe chest and back pain and shortness of breath. The onset of the pain was not sudden. He then launched into a lengthy monologue describing the origins of his pain. His descriptions were meticulous and precise, and his tone was unemotional and distant. Mr. Hall continued with his discourse, offering a detailed picture of a man whose current life had been severely affected by significant physical discomfort.

He had recently developed a pain that he believed to be a "cold" in his shoulder, which spread to his upper back. It became so severe he couldn't lie down in bed and would spend uncomfortable nights sitting or standing. When he developed a pain in his right calf, he called his doctor, who suggested taking aspirin for twenty-four hours and calling back if there was no improvement. The pain persisted and was soon followed by pains in his chest. When he finally visited his doctor, his regular internist, Dr. Brandon, was not in, and he was examined by Dr. Davis, another physician, who immediately focused on his leg. Mr. Hall neglected to emphasize his chest pain, since this regular doctor had already told him he'd scheduled a chest X ray as part of the visit. After going for the X ray, he returned to the doctor's office. There he saw Dr. Davis, who told him that the X ray was normal but that he had phlebitis, for which he was prescribed a medication.

The medicine did not relieve the pain, which remained severe. Mr. Hall called Dr. Davis and complained that his overriding problem was the chest pain, not the leg. Dr. Davis was surprised, since he had not been involved in any discussion of chest pain. He questioned Mr. Hall about shortness of breath, which the patient was experiencing, and prescribed a muscle relaxant.

Mr. Hall continued to deteriorate. His shortness of breath increased, and one day he coughed up some blood. Concerned about his new symptom, Mr. Hall called Dr. Brandon, his original doctor. Within half an hour Mr. Hall was checked into the hospital.

Mr. Hall's ability to protect himself from emotional distress was amazing. He was able to endure this extraordinary amount of suffering and pain—and to recount his story in so detached and calm a manner—because of his powers of denial. What is striking about Mr. Hall is the pervasiveness of his denial. He used many different maneuvers to ignore the presence of illness. He did admit he had heard it was possible to have phlebitis and develop blood clots in the chest when Richard Nixon suffered from phlebitis, but he "never imagined" that it would happen to him.

When Thomas Hall finally did seek medical attention, he still maintained a high level of denial by completely abdicating to his physicians the responsibility for recognizing and accurately assessing his physical impairment. His logic was simple: *I am sick only if my doctor finds something wrong.* This logic, however, is invalid if the patient distracts the physician from relevant signs and symptoms, and Mr. Hall was repeatedly guilty of doing exactly that.

It seems incredible that Mr. Hall could be unaware of the significance of his symptoms, particularly since he knew of Richard Nixon's much-publicized experience with phlebitis. He denied any connection between his physical condition and that of the former president by rationalizing that leg pain always precedes chest pain. Nonetheless, one would presume that he'd recognize that he had a serious illness of some sort. No cold could debilitate him so, yet during his ten days of symptoms he convinced himself that a cold was his only problem.

Mr. Hall had an *obsessional personality*, one that places a premium on intellect and rationality and minimizes the expression of feelings. He related his history mechanically, devoid of any emotion; he spoke from his head, not his heart. Mr. Hall is the type of person whose concern about events is muted by his ability to minimize his *feelings*. He accomplishes this by exaggerating his *intellectual understanding* of the issues at hand. Because he was threatened by his illness and its implications for his health and day-to-day functioning, he automatically utilized his standard psychological mechanisms to inhibit his emotional response. This allowed him to minimize serious symptoms, and he was therefore able to deny the existence of his phlebitis along with its potential impact on his life. When people like Mr. Hall contact their physicians, they must be taken very seriously: no matter how trivial the complaint, its significance can be extreme.

Case Study: Elizabeth Rader

Forty-one-year-old Elizabeth Rader was hospitalized for treatment of severe hypertension, a consequence of progressive kidney failure. She was born with a kidney malformation, which predisposed her to repeated infections since her youth. But she always ignored the impact of her illness. Like Thomas Hall, Ms. Rader recounted her medical history in extreme detail, and in a detached, intellectualized fashion, as though she were talking about someone else.

Ms. Rader had been treated for hypertension for almost twelve years. She had a kidney problem for at least thirty years. When younger, she experienced numerous comas with 104-degree fevers, cloudy urine, and days of continuous sleep. She suffered other symptoms such as extreme lethargy, fatigue, and pressure in the head. Symptoms would eventually disappear, but the disease progressed. She suffered extraordinary discomfort yet ignored her symptoms, attributing them to tiredness.

In contrast to Thomas Hall, Elizabeth Rader's long-standing denial suggested an impaired ability to differentiate between what is real and what is not. Her responses to the stress of illness revealed *massive denial*. Despite several kidney infections in her early life, she was never hospitalized. Despite the persistence of these episodes into college and graduate school, she was cared for only infrequently by a physician who was located in another city. She did not seek comprehensive, ongoing medical care because her infections "would usually go away by themselves" and because of her lack of medical insurance. This latter excuse became as flimsy as the first when it was learned that she came from a wealthy family. She coped with a significant health problem through an equally significant degree of denial. This attitude persisted even when she was suffering from side effects of the antihypertensive medication she was taking.

Elizabeth Rader shares several characteristics with Jeff Waldman and Thomas Hall. During her adolescence, she took the same omnipotent stance that Jeffrey Waldman did. Unconcerned about her several episodes of coma, she never sought treatment for this serious medical condition. In early adulthood, like Thomas Hall, she intellectualized and rationalized as a way of defending herself from emotional concerns caused by her illness. Her discussion of the various medications used to treat hypertension clearly illustrated this defensive style; she seemed considerably more interested in the pharmacologic nuances of these medicines than the physical effects of her damaged kidneys. Her denial, however, is different in character from that of the other two patients, because it continued for many years despite the persistence of obvious, serious physical symptoms. Ms. Rader's illness dynamics suggest reasons for this behavior.

Ms. Rader's family history is particularly telling. Her father, a medical researcher who did extensive experimentation with radiation, died of kidney cancer. The circumstances of her father's terminal illness left Ms. Rader resentful and distrustful of the medical profession. She felt that her father had developed cancer because of the profession's ignorance about radiation. She considered her father's surgeons inept, and implied that, had they been more technically skilled, her father would have survived the malignancy. She also felt that once surgery had failed to arrest the tumor, the profession had absolutely nothing to offer.

The parallels with her own illness are strong, including the fact that parent and child suffered from diseases of the same organ system. The profession was failing her in the same way it had failed her father by offering no hope for a cure. In sum, then, Elizabeth Rader felt destined to repeat her father's fate. Whether or not this fear was conscious, she dealt with her hopelessness by denying it completely. She conducted her life as if she were merely bothered by repeated colds rather than debilitated by progressive kidney failure.

Everyone exercises some denial at the onset of illness; as the first stage of the grief process, it provides a short-lived defense against the reality of ill health. However, if a person's illness dynamics promote maladaptive denial, it prevents healthy adaptation to illness and greatly complicates the task of health care providers. Unconscious rejection of the signs and symptoms of disease may impede efforts toward accurate diagnosis and comprehensive treatment. This can occur during any stage of illness, and it can produce a dangerous clinical situation. As illustrated by the preceding cases, prolonged denial can become self-destructive and possibly life threatening.

6

The Anxiety Response

Anxiety is at best an uncomfortable feeling. At its most extreme, anxiety can be a form of torture that prevents a person from carrying on normal day-to-day activities.

We all suffer from anxiety at some time; periodic, transient episodes are *common* responses to the events of daily life. A job interview or important test in school, for example, can provoke feelings of uncertainty and nervousness that are often augmented by such physical sensations as sweaty palms, churning stomach, or dry mouth. This completely normal emotional and physical response is known as *signal anxiety* because it actually prepares us to deal with stressful situations. Anxiety alerts us—and thereby helps us anticipate and cope with—particular stresses. This type of anxiety is positive, for it facilitates adaptation to the challenges encountered in daily life. In extreme circumstances—such as battle—it becomes essential for survival.

The degree of normal, adaptive anxiety is usually proportional to the intensity and type of stress that is felt. When anxiety becomes more intense, or longer in duration than warranted by a particular precipitating stress, it becomes *pathologic anxiety.* Such anxiety no longer serves the purpose of rousing the person; instead, it restricts functioning because its symptoms become excessive. Whereas a person suffering from anxiety is tense and uneasy, pathologic anxiety produces more pronounced feelings, such as fearfulness, marked agitation, and a sense of dread or foreboding. This is often accompanied by an increased sensitivity to external stimuli, so that even the sound of a ringing telephone can literally make the person jump. Focused concentration, or even just sitting still, may become difficult or impossible.

Physical distress is an integral part of pathologic anxiety. Common symptoms include: heart palpitations or rapid heartbeat; rapid breathing, often with shortness of breath and a choking sensation; dry mouth; gastrointestinal symptoms such as indigestion, nausea, vomiting, or diarrhea; and a generalized weakness. Some people develop specific bodily aches when anxious. Tension headaches, for example, can result from marked, sustained contraction of the muscles in the head and back of the neck. The physical symptoms accompanying a heightened state of anxiety reflect the general feeling of losing control. Many of these unpleasant bodily sensations are actually exaggerations of normal physiologic functions, such as rapid breathing. When the body goes into "overdrive" like this, people often worry that their biologic functioning will never return to normal. That fear, coupled with the generalized uneasiness of anxiety, raises concern about the ability to regain control over both emotions and body. People may also feel increasingly helpless as they anticipate and fear that loss of control. A vicious cycle can thus be perpetuated. Moreover, when handicapped by anxiety in this manner, people often become increasingly needy and dependent on relatives and close friends, who must take over some—or all—of their abdicated responsibilities. Whether the latter feel obligated, or compelled by their own sense of guilt, they too are ultimately burdened by the effects of someone else's pathologic anxiety.

We all feel anxious during the course of a physical illness, particularly at its onset. The appearance of a symptom—whether it is as ominous as persistent and unexplained weight loss, which may signal a progressing cancer, or as bothersome as nagging headaches—warns that the body is somehow not functioning properly. We wonder what is wrong and speculate about the seriousness of the problem. We worry about whether it is curable, or chronic, and anticipate what the diagnostic workup and ultimate treatment will entail. In the case of a serious illness, questions about the ongoing treatment can be cause for concern: Will my life-style be restricted for a while, or forever, by a special diet or decreased physical activity? What will be the impact of a lengthy illness and convalescence on my professional life? On family? On social relationships? What about financial considerations?

All this anxiety is a normal adjunct of disease. In fact, it is often an adaptive feeling, spurring a person to seek medical attention and then adhere to the prescribed treatment. The signal anxiety accompanying the onset of chest pain or the discovery of a lump in the breast warns that something is wrong and prompts the individual to do something about it. In a similar way, the recurrence of a symptom causes worry and concern in someone who is ill: anxiety that the disease is progressing prompts the patient to seek further medical care. Someone who does not feel anxious in these situations is denying normal concerns about illness, which could aggravate his or her physical problems. The recognition and acknowledgment of normal anxiety accompanying physical illness ultimately results in better medical treatment and, it is hoped, an improved prognosis.

Medical illness can also precipitate pathologic anxiety. When that happens, patients become overly concerned about their physical status. The anxiety that subsequently occurs is much more severe or lasts much longer than is usually warranted by their particular disease. Pathologic anxiety is clearly an abnormal response to illness, one with potentially dangerous ramifications. When a person is overcome with anxiety about an illness, other emotions are overshadowed by the anxiety and assume a secondary, and possibly negligible, role in the psychological adjustment to sickness. This results in an inability to properly grieve the loss of health and come to an acceptance of ill health.

People who suffer from pathologic anxiety about their illness tend to become hypersensitive to all aspects of medical treatment. The main focus of their daily lives is a preoccupation with any alteration of bodily function; a new ache takes on tremendous significance, regardless of how trivial or transient it may be. One consequence of this kind of anxiety is an impaired ability to provide an accurate medical history. For example, minor muscle pains, which a person previously ignored, may now become incorporated into an increasingly distorted assessment of health. This person may repeatedly call the doctor to report these new findings, despite assurances that there is no need for concern. In addition, the physical symptoms that accompany anxiety may be difficult to distinguish from symptoms attributable to the patient's disease.

Excessive anxiety can also cause a patient to experience every diagnostic test, every change in medication or diet, every treatment, and every visit to the doctor as portents of danger. That is, he or she ruminates about *why* the doctor prescribed another pill, or ordered another blood test, convinced that it is an ominous sign of the progression of ill health. Or the patient is unremittingly apprehensive about an additional X ray, certain that it is a signal he or she is rapidly succumbing to the disease. Such pathologic anxiety can cause patients to view medical personnel as the enemy—the bearers of sad tidings, rather than as dispensers of hope. This can disrupt a collaborative doctor-patient relationship, with serious consequences for overall treatment. For example, a woman may become so fearful that she simply refuses to pursue further medical care. Or, on the other hand, she may seek constant reassurance to calm her fears: this unrelenting request for support may aggravate her caretakers, making them less sensitive or caring in their work with her.

Case Study: Laura Levine

Thirty-year-old Laura Levine has a career, is married, and has a nine-year-old son. Eight years before her meeting with the therapist, she went to the Emergency Room to be examined for flulike symptoms. The diagnosis was sarcoidosis, a chronic disease of unknown cause that is similar to tuberculosis.

Sarcoidosis produces inflammation in the tissue of many organs of the body, causing such symptoms as swollen lymph glands, difficulty in breathing, enlargement of the liver, spleen, or salivary glands, skin lesions, and inflammation of the eyes. In addition, the patient may experience low-grade fever, fatigue, weight loss, weakness, and generalized malaise. The clinical course of the disease varies greatly from one patient to another. Although it is usually benign, with some asymptomatic patients getting diagnosed only through incidental X-ray findings, it can potentially cause severe incapacity and even death.

Sarcoidosis is a somewhat mysterious disease. Not only is there uncertainty over its cause, but its clinical course is unpredictable. Although most patients undergo a complete spontaneous remission with no evidence of disease, some have persistent physical abnormalities with varying degrees of disability, and others experience progressive deterioration and incapacitation. When diagnosed with the disease, the patient is usually told that he or she has a chronic illness with an erratic course that may be characterized by acute flare-ups interspersed with periods of remission. Thus, whereas the doctor can assure the patient that any medical treatment provided will be appropriate and thorough, the doctor cannot specify precisely what the treatment will be until the disease demonstrates its involvement with one or more organs—if it does so at all.

The uncertainty of sarcoidosis makes it difficult to cope

with emotionally. Someone in remission may totally deny any concerns about possible progression of the disease, whereas others, like Laura Levine, become so worried about the potential danger of sarcoidosis that their preoccupation becomes the major aspect of their lives. Although she might have reacted better to an illness with a more predictable prognosis, Ms. Levine's particular illness dynamics greatly aggravated her emotional response to sarcoidosis. Her chronic worry infringed on her family life, her career, and her relationship with health care providers.

Her disease was initially diagnosed back in 1970, when she went to the Emergency Room to have pains in her chest and side checked out. Although the initial diagnosis was pneumonia, the Emergency Room doctor called her the next day and referred her to another physician, who made the preliminary diagnosis of sarcoidosis, pending the results of a biopsy of her lymph node. The doctor prescribed medication for her illness, which caused a rash that required treatment, including more medication. She then repeatedly experienced chest pains of such severity that she had to keep going to the Emergency Room, but the doctors couldn't find anything wrong with her.

After a year, Ms. Levine went to another doctor for a complete physical. He diagnosed a "nervous condition"—that is, chronic anxiety—and prescribed tranquilizers for her. She took the medication "for a while and started getting a little better," but she resisted taking the tranquilizers regularly, because, even though they made her feel better, she believed they were "the wrong medication for sarcoidosis." Despite her doctor's repeated assurances that her disease was in remission and that her frequent complaints were most probably due to gastrointestinal symptoms, Ms. Levine feared that the sarcoidosis was progressing rapidly.

Her husband grew increasingly distressed, recognizing that his wife had been dramatically transformed by her illness. Previously a highly responsible woman who balanced a taxing professional career with the demands of motherhood, Ms. Levine had become emotionally debilitated, anxious, and helpless—far beyond what the course of her disease would seem to suggest.

In 1982 Ms. Levine visited yet another doctor for a repeat physical examination. He also diagnosed a nervous condition. However, Ms. Levine remained skeptical, because her various pains had not disappeared completely. She could not understand the need for tranquilizers—even though they made her feel better. Her refusal to believe that her persisting symptoms were related to gastrointestinal problems was particularly surprising, given her earlier medical history. She used to have digestive problems in the tenth grade. A doctor gave her a complete physical and told her mother she had "nervous indigestion" and prescribed some medication that cleared it up. Later, when she got pregnant, she again had indigestion, for nine months, and then it disappeared.

Laura Levine confided to the therapist that even though she was always in great pain when she set out for the hospital, she started to feel better by the time she entered the Emergency Room—before she was examined by a doctor or given any medications. She also stated that she was never completely satisfied with the explanation that her pains were due to indigestion as opposed to sarcoidosis.

The intense anxiety Ms. Levine felt about her disease pervaded every aspect of her life. Sometimes when she and her husband went out for the evening, they would have to go home early because she would "start hurting." Sometimes she wasn't able to do things like go to the gym or socialize with friends because her chest hurt. She continued working but felt "miserable" when she was at the office.

Many physicians had told Ms. Levine that the disease could have a favorable course. However, despite their reenforcement, she could not rid herself of the panicked notion that the sarcoidosis was advancing inexorably, crippling her body. She might visit the Emergency Room two or three nights a week, for months at a time, complaining of countless nonspecific symptoms that she feared were related to the sarcoidosis. Those varied symptoms persisted even though many physicians told her they could find no evidence of *any* disease and also explained that sarcoidosis often goes into remission for long periods and may even disappear after the initial episode. None of this reassured her. Ms. Levine's pathologic anxiety caused her to lose all perspective when assessing her body's functioning.

Laura Levine's complaints are symptoms of chronic anxiety, which her doctors recognized. That is why they prescribed tranquilizers and antacid medication, which have no effect on sarcoidosis but provide temporary relief from anxiety symptoms. During her many visits to the Emergency Room, she reported the presence of common signs of chronic anixety: rapid heartbeat, profuse sweating, rapid breathing with a choked feeling, and a "scared" feeling. She demonstrated the pervasive nagging apprehension, uneasiness, and doubt that characterize abnormal anxiety. Repeated trips to at least five different doctors only produced the same diagnosis each time: "a nervous condition." These visits provided her with constant reassurance against her dreaded fantasy that the sarcoidosis had become more serious and severe. The fact that her pain vanished while she waited for a physician to examine her suggests that the safety of a hospital environment allayed her anxiety; as it diminished, her stomach pains disappeared. Unfortunately, Ms. Levine's anxiety was so great that she was never fully able to accept the reassurance of the doctors who informed her that she was in complete remission.

Why did she consistently refuse to believe what should have been good news from her doctors? Her family history provided answers to this question. Her mother had tuberculosis and was hospitalized for nine months with the disease in 1960. Initially, the doctors had misdiagnosed her illness, calling it pneumonia. At about the same time, her sister died suddenly of a blood clot in her lungs, leaving behind three children, including a month-old baby, and a husband. Ms. Levine moved in with her sister's family to help out with the children. About a week after her mother was hospitalized, her father also entered the hospital, suffering from fluid in his leg. Ms. Levine was left to carry the whole family.

Her father was released from the hospital after about four weeks and was doing well until several years later, when he developed recurrent problems with kidney stones and underwent three or four operations. He also had a heart problem. When he died, the doctors attributed it to a heart attack, but Ms. Levine noted it came right after an operation for his kidney stones. This interpretation left her with some strong feelings about her own medical condition and care.

Ms. Levine's background and her family's medical history brought her illness dynamics into focus and suggested why she experienced an anxiety response to ill health. There is evidence that she reacts to any stress with anxiety. Her "nervous stomach" earlier in her life was probably an anxiety symptom, first diagnosed during a predictably difficult developmental period. She was then a young adolescent, struggling with the confusing issues of that time of life. Her gastrointestinal symptoms reflected her emotional response to this period and signaled the potential for anxiety as a characteristic style—a kind of patterned response—of reacting to stress.

The nature of her illness was an additional stressor. Sarcoidosis *is* a puzzling disease, characterized by both clinical remissions, in which all evidence of the disease can disappear, and an ever-present potential for flare-ups. This type of illness allows the patient the option of either gratefully accepting a remission and relaxing or anxiously anticipating a relapse. Ms. Levine habitually chose the latter course, a reaction dictated by her illness dynamics.

In all probability, the most significant aspect of Ms. Levine's case history—the one that had the greatest effect on her own response to illness—was her perception of the medical treatment her family had received over the years. In recounting her history to the therapist, she revealed a pervasive mistrust of physicians, who, she felt, attributed all her physical symptoms to nerves. The initial incorrect diagnosis of her mother's tuberculosis, the alleged mismanagement of her father's condition, which is linked in her mind with his death, and the sudden death of a young, healthy sister after the birth of her baby all contributed to Ms. Levine's strong emotional response to her illness.

Ms. Levine, like her mother, was misdiagnosed when her problem first appeared. And ironically, her illness was similar to her mother's, also producing symptoms in her lungs. It is reasonable to suspect that this caused Ms. Levine considerable worry about the thoroughness and effectiveness of her treatment. More than likely, it also triggered fears about whether she would get sicker and require lengthy medical treatment, as her mother did, or even share the tragic fate of her sister and die suddenly at an early age. Her father's medical treatment further diminished Ms. Levine's faith in physicians. She sincerely believed that the kidney-stone operation had killed him, and that his physician had been both ignorant and negligent. This view corresponded to her feelings about the effects of her own biopsy—the one that confirmed her diagnosis of sarcoidosis. She stated that her recurrent chest pain had worsened since her "operation," even though the procedure itself is benign and relatively painless. Although it is possible that the biopsy was the cause of her recurrent chest pain, such an outcome is highly unlikely. The biopsy probably provoked anxiety by affirming the presence of a chronic disease. Her emotional discomfort was expressed as a common anxiety symptom (recurrent, nonspecific aches and pains, which she herself attributed to a physical problem). Given her conviction that physicians had mistreated her family—in her mind causing them pain, suffering, even death—she was ready to attribute some of her own suffering to the ineptitude of her physicians as evidenced, for example, by a poorly performed biopsy.

Laura Levine's abnormal concern for her health was tragic. She was crippled, a prisoner of her own anxiety. Not only did she suffer from the discomfort of annoying symptoms, anxiety also interfered with every aspect of her life. In reality, her sarcoidosis had already been in remission for three years and had become a secondary problem in her life. Her primary illness was her emotional response to sarcoidosis. Sadly, Ms. Levine felt that the prospects for her adapting to and resolving her feelings were not hopeful. When asked how she thought she would be feeling in the future, she replied: "About the way I'm doing now. I think if nothing changes and they can't really find anything wrong with me—something has to be serious—I know I'll be having these digestive problems. I'll probably be taking tranquilizers off and on continually."

Adaptive anxiety promotes positive behaviors that help maintain health. It provides the motivation to practice preventive care, such as scheduling immunizations and adhering to a healthy diet, as well as to seek timely medical attention following the onset of symptoms. Its persistence during an episode of ill health, secondary to concerns about such diverse issues as the discomfort of diagnostic procedures or physical limitations to daily functioning, further motivates compliance with treatment.

When anxiety becomes excessive, when the concerns it causes far outweigh its protective function, it promotes an irrational preoccupation with health issues that may evolve into a pathologic illness response. In this circumstance patients react as Laura Levine did and become hypersensitive to all aspects of an illness. Such hypersensitivity greatly detracts from all other aspects of life, progressively displacing good feelings with a debilitating *angst*. Paradoxically, it also interferes with medical care. Heightened anxiety compromises objectivity and, consequently, ability to provide an accurate history, tolerate certain diagnostic procedures, or even cooperate in a routine physical exam. Should this progress into chronic anxiety, the patient is then burdened with an unpleasant, counterproductive emotional state, along with the limitations caused by the physical problem. In addition, continued demands for reassurance from friends, family, and health care personnel may progressively alienate those support systems. In this fashion, the anxiety response compromises diverse aspects of medical treatment and thus diminishes the chances for returning to full health or achieving an optimal level of functioning given the nature of the illness.

7

The Anger Response

Anger is one of the emotions accompanying loss. Failing at some endeavor or losing the car keys might provoke mild annoyance or frustration, whereas life crises of greater consequence—such as getting divorced or being fired from a job—produce more intense and sustained hostility. When circumstances conspire to take from us something or someone we cherish, we always feel angry.

The same feelings accompany illness: we are angry when we lose our health. This is as true for a simple upper respiratory infection as it is for a more serious or chronic illness, though of course the circumstances of the disease dictate the degree of anger that is felt. Upon awaking one morning to the pain of a scratchy throat or congested sinuses, early signs of an upper respiratory infection, a person feels annoyed and anticipates several days of unpleasant symptoms. Memories of previous episodes may recur, especially if the earlier illness was marked by particular discomfort.

Whereas an upper respiratory infection is inconvenient, causing only transitory feelings of irritation, a more serious illness may cause feelings of extreme anger, with more pronounced expressions of hostility toward other people.

Bob King is a nineteen-year-old who had suffered a traumatic amputation of his foot as the result of a hit-and-run auto accident the previous year. He was hospitalized for treatment of osteomyelitis, a bone infection that had been present since the accident. Loss of a limb is always difficult to cope with, and Mr. King's case was particularly tragic, for he had been a superb athlete and held a football scholarship to a major university. He had looked forward to a successful athletic career as a means of escaping a difficult family situation and a marginal socioeconomic position. His shattered limb seemed to symbolize his shattered future.

The degree of Mr. King's rage was extreme, and the intensity of his fury was frightening. He threatened to "get even" with the driver of the other car, who had caused the accident by running a stop sign and then fled without offering assistance. He was bitter toward his girlfriend, who was drifting from their relationship because he was "a cripple," and angry with his "useless" physicians who were unable to halt the infection.

Mr. King's anger was not confined to the person who had caused his accident; he was angry at everybody. His physicians, his girlfriend, and visitors to his hospital room were targets for his rage. This diffuse hostility is an important aspect of the anger response to illness. Aggression is manifested in several directions—toward oneself, toward family and friends, toward physicians and other health care personnel, toward the Fates—and is rarely confined to a single area. In this regard, the anger response to illness is reminiscent of the anger phase of normal grief. However, unlike grief, it is characterized by sustained, intense hostility so pronounced that it prevents the patient from recognizing and expressing any other emotions. In effect, the patient is *mad rather than sad*, which inhibits the progression of normal grief.

Four Targets of Anger

In the anger response, there are four target areas for hostility. *Global anger* is a diffuse, nonspecific hostility directed at no one person in particular. Many patients feel cheated and angry about the unfairness of illness. They ask "Why me?" and feel angry when they realize there is no satisfactory answer to that question. This is particularly true when they have responsibly attended to their health. Unfortunately, life isn't always fair, and the indiscriminate onset of illness makes people angry.

As an illness progresses, some people become *angry with themselves*. This may be expressed overtly, with demeaning, self-deprecating talk, or passively through masochistic behavior, such as neglecting necessary treatment. There are several explanations for this kind of behavior. Some people feel great responsibility for their ailments, believing they caused a sickness by excesses, such as overeating or smoking. This is especially true if they have disregarded warnings from family or physicians or minimized symptoms of ill health. Patients may also become angry at themselves because of the decreased autonomy that accompanies some kinds of illness. Some people simply hate getting older: an episode of illness can remind them of their own mortality, which they find difficult to accept. They frequently become disgusted when something—no matter how trivial—goes wrong with their bodies. Finally, anger can become self-directed when illness interferes with the pursuit of a long-cherished dream. If a middle-age man planned to travel later in life, for instance, he may become infuriated with himself for postponing this activity, if illness now makes it an impossibility.

Some patients *take their anger out on those closest to them*. They may resent family and friends simply because they are not ill and don't have to contend with the consequences of ill health. To some degree, the patient might even perceive his or her loved ones as outsiders who do not understand the meaning of being sick. The patient may also resent other family members if the illness upsets the family equilibrium and thereby alters established roles. For example, the usually dependent family member may be forced into a more active, assertive position if illness prevents the wage earner from continued employment. This can provoke significant resentment in someone who, already stressed by diminished autonomy, feels threatened by the new independence of his or her spouse. Sometimes people also blame family members for their illness. They feel that another family member aggravated them excessively or was even the cause of their unhealthy habits or life-styles.

People also blame their families by becoming angry at ancestors for passing on a poor genetic heritage. Statements such as "I knew I'd have a heart attack early in my life because everyone in my father's family died that way before age fifty" reflect this kind of hostility. Even if the patient doesn't suffer a heart attack, any symptom suggestive of heart disease, such as hypertension, is all the more frightening to him or her. When a person feels afraid, he or she usually feels angry toward those he or she believes are responsible for the fear—in the case, those who passed on to their children and grandchildren a predilection toward a specific disease.

In addition, people who are influenced by their family's medical history frequently identify with ancestors who suffered through a specific illness. As a result, they can think of a particular illness only in terms of the exact effects it had upon their family member. For example, Tom Shore's grandfather became blind as a result of his diabetes. When Mr. Shore was diagnosed with diabetes, he was certain it meant that he, too, would go blind, even though not everyone who gets diabetes loses his or her sight. Mr. Shore became resentful of his grandfather for passing on his "defective gene" and for making him aware of the devastating impact of the disease. Unfortunately, Mr. Shore did not realize that his view of diabetes was distorted, reflecting only one potential outcome of his own illness.

Physicians and health care personnel are often the targets of a patient's anger, which may be conscious or unconscious and range from mild irritation to extreme hostility. This is due, in part, to the fact that physicians are often the bearers of sad—and unwelcome—tidings. Many patients also resent the degree of control physicians exercise over them. A doctor can commit a patient to a hospital and then further disrupt his or her life with diagnostic procedures and therapeutic regimens that may be embarrassing, painful, debilitating, or disfiguring. Doctors impose dietary restrictions, dictate acceptable levels of activity, and prescribe medications that may have unpleasant side effects. All this is done with the implicit (and sometimes explicit) message that the patient has no choice but to accede to these requirements if he or she is to improve. By its very nature, the doctor-patient relationship fosters a hostile dependency, which enrages those who resent the loss of autonomy that follows the onset of illness. In addition, doctors are stereotypically perceived as fit and healthy—incapable of empathizing with the patient's ill health. Many physicians hear patients report, "You don't understand what I'm going through because you don't have arthritis." That perceived lack of empathy can also foster anger in an already debilitated patient.

Everyone responds to illness with some anger and directs it toward these four targets. However, unlike the anger phase of normal grief, the anger response to illness is characterized by hostility so pronounced in degree and prolonged in duration that it overshadows the expression of any other emotions accompanying the illness. In this kind of response, the patient's angry feelings do not gradually subside and make way for depressed feelings, the next stage of grief. The anger perpetuates itself and becomes more intense over time. Bob King's tragedy illustrates this dramatically. A year after his accident, he still exhibited a diffuse, treacherous rage. He had not even started to feel the sadness associated with the loss of his limb; his anger was more comfortable to him than the depressing reality concerning his lost athletic career. This interfered with the normal grief process and prevented him from coming to terms with his loss so that he could proceed with his life.

Case Study: Nellie Thomas

Nellie Thomas, a seventy-three-year-old with a long history of arthritis, was hospitalized with a swollen and tender knee after a fall in her backyard. She was accustomed to inflamed joints, resulting from her chronic arthritis, and despite this illness had lived an extremely active life. An avid traveler since her twenties, she was a true adventurer who not only had explored the world's outposts, but had also written several books about her exploits. She initially thought her recent fall had caused a flare-up of her illness, but diagnostic tests revealed an infected knee. She had a staphylococcal infection that was surgically drained and treated with intravenous antibiotics. However, this treatment did not contain the infection—which spread through her bloodstream and caused an endocarditis, an inflammation of her heart valves, which left her gravely ill for several weeks. She was only able to begin to contemplate discharge from the hospital approximately three months following her admission.

Nellie Thomas acted like a petulant child in expressing her feelings about her accident and treatment. She was sarcastic and demeaning with staff and visitors. She communicated her anger in a negativistic, passive manner and frequently sulked in silence. She found her medical treatment painful and agonizing. Her contempt for her medical caregivers was also inspired by an idealized view of her father, a "famous" surgeon from the Yale School of Medicine who "never submitted a patient to unnecessary pain."

Nellie's anger was focused toward one target: the medical profession. Instead of voicing self-recriminations about her fall or cursing the Fates for her ill fortune, she relentlessly demeaned those caring for her—doctors, nurses, and physical therapists. She condemned her care-givers as ineffectual, sadistic people who derived pleasure from inflicting pain. There are several reasons for this jaundiced view.

Since Ms. Thomas was an avid traveler, confinement of any kind—especially the regimented hospital routine—was torture for her. She was also enraged at her help-lessness and furious about the time wasted because of her illness. Moreover, she considered her treatment incompetent and therefore the greatest obstacle to her liberation from the hospital. Despite surgical and med-ical interventions, her infection had progressed to life-threatening proportions. In her view, not only had the doctors confined her, they had also caused her more pain and suffering, allowed her to become increasingly debili-tated, and prolonged her convalescence at a period in her life when time was especially precious. She felt righteous indignation toward the medical community and justified in her fury.

The other strong determinant to Nellie Thomas's anger response derived from her perception of her father. In her mind none of the efforts of her current doctors could com-pare with his humanism and efforts to spare his patients unnecessary pain. She idolized her father, and hence no physician could compete with him. They all disappointed her; they were all objects of ridicule when compared with her renowned father. Her past experiences and perceptions of her father prevented an objective assessment of her pres-ent caretakers. If her physicians had failed to realize these origins of her anger, if they had personalized her attacks, their relationship with her would have quickly deterio-rated into a useless struggle that would have seriously interfered with her treatment. Fortunately they under-stood the underlying motivations of her behavior, and this understanding allowed them to remain objective and em-pathically concerned with her treatment despite her fre-quent criticism and abuse.

Case Study: Janet Roper

Janet Roper, a sixty-seven-year-old, has a ten-year history of cardiovascular disease. When she initially consulted her doctor for intermittent angina, she was diagnosed as having high blood pressure and given treatment that kept the condition under control. However, seven years ago she suffered a stroke which left her partially paralyzed. Her impaired functioning forced her to leave a factory job she had held for twenty-two years. She became financially dependent on medical disability payments and had to rely on the assistance of a housekeeper. Despite her obvious impairment, she adjusted to her ill health, continuing her volunteer work for her church and traveling often to visit family and friends.

The first time Ms. Roper was rehospitalized was five years following her stroke, when she had a heart attack while in another city. She recovered from the acute illness, but her angina continued to become more severe, increasing in frequency and intensity until she required daily doses of nitroglycerin. During the two years following her heart attack she was hospitalized three times with the same complaint of intractable angina. Each time she was admitted to the hospital because her physicians felt that her symptoms signaled another heart attack. Each time she obtained symptomatic relief, only to have the pain recur at her usual level of discomfort when she returned home. Although she never actually suffered another heart attack, Ms. Roper was extremely displeased with her treatment because her anginal pain continued.

Janet Roper's response to her long-standing health problems was a pervasive, sustained anger. She condemned her family for not supporting her, criticized her physicians for not curing her, and even cursed God for abandoning her despite her deep religious convictions. In her mind, it was a simple matter: no one had successfully relieved the pain stemming from her angina, and for that she was unforgiving.

Ms. Roper's anger response to her heart attack and continuing angina contrasted sharply with her apparent adjustment to the earlier stroke. This was due to the fact that despite some residual paralysis, her condition after the stroke was relatively stable and permitted a certain degree of autonomy. The heart attack, on the other hand, resulted in chronic, unstable angina that was painful and unpredictable. Her life was much less under her own control. Lack of control was an important reason for her anger response, but not the major reason.

A look at Ms. Roper's relationship with her parents provides a clue to understanding her illness response. Her mother was "mean," and to defy her invited ostracism or physical harm. These perceptions may have been exaggerated, but they still shaped Ms. Roper's feelings toward nurturing and authority: compliance is rewarded, disobedience severely punished. Her earliest experiences taught her to respond to authority with terror—and subsequently fury. This response established a conventional wisdom for her, and it prevailed throughout her life. Her interactions with physicians exemplified these dynamics. Completely accepting of their authority, she was comfortable with her passivity when treatment was successful. However, when the doctors were unable to relieve her symptoms, she felt cheated because they failed to reward her compliance. This enraged her, but she was too fearful to criticize them openly. Instead, her anger was expressed as a smoldering resentment; the powerful legacy of a domineering mother was acted out in her continuing resentment of control.

Janet Roper idealized her father, describing him as the one person she loved. She poignantly illustrated the intense pain she suffered after his death with a simple statement: "The day he died, I died." Turning toward religion, she transferred to God some feelings she held for her own father. Just as she looked to her father for support and protection from her mother, she frequently turned to God for guidance, strength, and relief during periods of illness. Ms. Roper's statement "I'm going to fight God from now on" was surprising, but understandable in light of her feelings that Jesus had abandoned her. She came to this conclusion because, in spite of her faithful worship, her suffering continued unabated. The parallel to her feelings at the time of her father's death is clear. On that occasion, her sadness was accompanied by considerable anger, for she depended on her father for support against her mother's wrath. The rage she had been able to contain until now by expression of faith finally emerged when she concluded that God, like her biologic father, had abandoned her.

The hallmark of the anger response is *conflict,* which is communicated through words or deed, either overtly or covertly. Instead of working through feelings fostered by an illness, the patient engages in a variety of struggles with the people in his or her life. These may be obvious, such as debate surrounding a refusal to submit to a diagnostic procedure or consent to rehabilitative therapy. The impotent pleas of family members urging reconsideration, as well as the frustration of health care providers, reflect the patient's considerable hostility. Covert struggles can take the form of *passive-aggression,* such as ignoring dietary restrictions or irresponsibly adhering to a medication regimen, behaviors that afford the patient the pleasure of secret control over his or her caretakers. *Displacement* is an additional means of disguising anger about the loss of health, as the hostility is transferred to other life circumstances. For example, the recurrence of old marital disputes permits the expression of anger without directly identifying illness as its root cause.

In sum, the anger response promotes a generalized noncompliance with treatment, progressively transforming the patient's supportive alliances—including those with caretakers—into adversarial relationships. In addition to detracting from the level of medical care, this reaction often isolates the patient from a support system that could provide help in negotiating the stressful life situation of ill health.

8

The Depression Response

The word *depression* is generally overused—and often used incorrectly. Depression is not the expression of the normal sadness that accompanies difficult life circumstances. The expression of such sadness, as discussed in Chapter 3, is an integral part of grief and is necessary for coping adequately with a loss. Someone in the throes of a typical grief response does, in fact, feel many of the same emotions as a person suffering from depression, but there is a difference. Depression is pathologic: it is a disease. And, like any other disease, depression has specific signs and symptoms that define its diagnosis and course. Although it is categorized as an emotional disorder, depression, like any other disease, affects both the mind and the body.

The diagnosis of depression involves four major categories of symptoms. First, *depression is characterized by changes in emotional state*, usually in an ongoing lowering of mood. At best, the depressed individual is subdued; someone more severely depressed may feel profound sadness punctuated by frequent bouts of tearfulness and crying. The joy of living has disappeared for such people. As the sense of despair grows, so does the sense of loneliness and isolation. Suicidal thoughts and behavior may follow. Alternatively, depression sometimes involves elevation of mood. Some individuals become chronically anxious or agitated, feeling incapable of relaxation. In extreme cases manic feelings, even euphoria, predominate. Although these feelings might appear contradictory to a depressed state, they may actually be an unconscious defense that serves to distract from the pain of a profound underlying sadness.

The second category of changes induced by depression is physiologic. Bodily changes are varied and affect many different organs. Perhaps the most common physiologic change associated with depression is a disturbance in sleeping patterns. Many people suffering from the illness report either difficulty falling asleep, waking frequently during the night, waking up early in the morning and being unable to fall back asleep, or sleeping excessively. A diminished energy level, often accompanied by lethargy, listlessness, and chronic fatigue, is associated with these sleep disturbances. Some people suffer from difficulty in concentrating, experiencing memory lapses or a more generalized forgetfulness. The sex drive may be impaired, resulting in decreased interest in sexual activity or diminished enjoyment and pleasure. Often, a woman's menstrual cycle becomes irregular or even ceases for several months. In short, there are numerous kinds of physical ailments that may appear when someone is depressed. These may be nonspecific, such as vague muscular aches and pains, or more focused, such as the headaches or lower back pain frequently reported by depressed patients. Whatever the complaint, one thing remains consistent for all people suffering from depression: the illness has a pervasive impact on the normal physical functioning of the body.

The third category of symptoms experienced by depressed people is a progressive lowering of self-esteem. This may be a reaction to changes in mood and impaired mental and physical functioning. Fearing the external loss of the former self, the depressed person becomes plagued with self-doubt, and the self-image turns harshly negative. Common feelings are those of weakness, guilt, helplessness, and worthlessness. In fact, this damage to self-esteem may bring feelings of hopelessness and cause the depression to deepen.

The fourth major aspect of depression is an alteration of the usual patterns of behavior. The most common change is a generalized withdrawal—both emotionally and physically—from the environment. Depression can cause feelings of inferiority, which enhance a sense of detachment from others. It can also cause a loss of interest in daily activities—family, relationships, work, recreation, and social functions—which serves to further isolate the depressed individual. As interest in daily life wanes, so does the ability to perform everyday functions. The world becomes a boring, joyless, and threatening place: an increasing amount of time is spent alone. Long solitary walks, much time spent reading or watching television, or even sleeping for many hours each day are hallmarks of depression. Everyday behavior becomes severely limited by this lack of enjoyment in life and alienation from the world. As a result, the depression deepens.

Elements of each of these four interrelated components must be present for a physician to make a diagnosis of depression. Much like grieving, depression affects the body, the emotions, perceptions of both oneself and one's environment, and the conduct of one's daily life. Depression, however, can be differentiated from normal grief by means of two distinguishing factors: *degree* and *purpose.* Grief is a dynamic growth process, during which a person reminisces about what he or she has lost, recalling the associated positive and negative emotions. By acknowledging and analyzing the feelings related to a loss, the bereaved can establish a new emotional equilibrium and continue to get satisfaction and pleasure from life. Depression, on the other hand, interferes with the enjoyment of life. Unlike a normal grief response, depression brings stagnation, not growth. Generally, the symptoms of depression are more severe, last longer, and interfere more profoundly with normal functioning.

Numerous hypotheses have been raised regarding the mechanisms responsible for depression. Current scientific belief posits both a biological and an emotional component to depression. Widespread investigation during the past two decades demonstrates that disorders of mood are often caused by an imbalance of certain chemicals in the brain. Such biologic dysfunction is definitely implicated in depression, as proven by laboratory experiments in which drugs administered to lab animals depleted their brains of specific substances, resulting in objective signs and symptoms of depression. There is also overwhelming evidence that exclusively psychologic events can produce depression. For example, British psychiatrist Rene Spitz observed that infants deprived of sufficient maternal care and nurturing withdrew from their external environments, became progressively debilitated by their depression, and ultimately died.

Unquestionably, depression involves an interplay of biological and psychological events. Although it is usually impossible to determine whether one or the other component is cause or effect, there are some instances where the cause-and-effect relationship is clear-cut. For example, the widespread prevalence of manic-depressive illness in a family indicates genetic transmission of the disease. The depression caused by loss of health, on the other hand, derives from an inability to acknowledge fully and to put into perspective all the emotions relating to a particular loss.

Case Study: Carl Nunez

Carl Nunez, a seventy-five-year-old taxi driver, was admitted to the hospital following a fainting spell that had been accompanied by severe pain in the chest and left shoulder. It was subsequently determined that Mr. Nunez had suffered a heart attack. During the first twenty-four hours in the hospital, his blood pressure dropped and there was concern that he was going into shock. Insertion of a temporary pacemaker quickly stabilized his condition. The physicians were pleased with his progress; he showed remarkable physical resilience for a man of his age. However, his emotional adaptation to his illness was not as good.

As early as the second day of his hospitalization, according to the nursing notes, Mr. Nunez became "belligerent and aggravated . . . stating that he doesn't want to be here and he would rather die." Several days later a nurse reported "the patient feels fine physically but says he has felt for a while that his life has been long enough." Ironically, as he became stronger physically, he became increasingly debilitated emotionally. He complained of lethargy, chronic fatigue, anorexia, and poor concentration, and he was frequently observed to be tearful or crying. While the lowering of his physical and mental energy levels could be at least partly attributed to his heart attack, Mr. Nunez was unquestionably depressed. His clinical depression was a greater threat to his well-being than his heart condition. As a result, approximately three weeks after his admission he was transferred to an inpatient psychiatric unit for treatment.

When he met with the therapist, Mr. Nunez looked like a beaten man. He was unkempt; his clothes, wrinkled and dirty, hung from his body, indicating weight loss. He wasn't wearing socks, and his shoes were untied. He obviously hadn't shaved in days. He sat almost motionless on the edge of his bed, shoulders hunched over, head hanging down, staring at the floor. When answering questions, he moved and spoke slowly, his voice very soft. He seemed distracted, periodically drifting off and staring into space.

Mr. Nunez was clearly upset by the acute illness; his concerns, coupled with insecurity about his future, caused him to become depressed. He described some of the common symptoms—loss of appetite, tiredness, unexplained crying—then talked of his major fear concerning the illness.

Mr. Nunez had been driving a cab more than forty-eight years. After his heart attack, he didn't believe he would be able to return to work. He admitted to feeling sad. The sadness confused him, because, as he said repeatedly, he really had "nothing to be sad about." While he was aware that this overwhelming sadness started right after his heart attack, he was not able to explain the connection between the two.

Mr. Nunez's symptoms meet three of the four criteria for depression. His mood was profoundly sad, punctuated by a good deal of crying. He reported common physical symptoms characteristic of depression: lack of appetite with weight loss, fatigue, lack of energy, and difficulty sleeping. His self-esteem was markedly impaired. This negativism was particularly apparent when he speculated about his future—he imagined he would be incapable of doing anything. The fourth aspect of depression, changes in established behavior patterns, could only be inferred because Mr. Nunez had not yet returned to his usual environment. However, it was observed that he was becoming increasingly isolated from patients and staff on the ward. This behavior, combined with his fears about being unable to carry out his daily activities upon leaving the hospital, suggested movement toward a more generalized withdrawal from his environment.

It was difficult to imagine that only a month earlier he had been a vigorous, energetic man, a responsible provider for his family who had joyful enthusiasm for work and recreation. His heart attack had obviously precipitated his depression: his sadness began, in his words, "the day I got sick." But why did he become so overwhelmed by his illness that he required inpatient psychiatric treatment? The answer is obvious when considering the psychological components of his illness dynamics.

Mr. Nunez was a survivor. His independence and self-sufficiency enabled him to provide for himself and his family for more than sixty years. He accepted the challenges that came his way and survived by means of his native intelligence and common sense. Mr. Nunez's personality was strongly devoted to obtaining and maintaining control of his life. Not to be in control of his life was anathema to him, and that was precisely what happened after his heart attack.

Mr. Nunez's self-sufficiency was undermined from the very beginning of his illness, which literally struck him down. He could not comprehend his helplessness. The initial belligerence reported by the nursing staff was his attempt to regain some semblance of control over his life, even while desperately ill. This protest was born of the fear that came from his self-perception: he was a sick man, and his illness posed a threat to his way of life. He tried to deal with the fear in characteristic fashion—through action—but his physical condition prevented him from doing so. Never having been ill before, he had not developed alternative coping skills to help him adjust to being sick. Furthermore, he was unable to view his heart attack with any perspective; he could not appreciate that he had progressed well physically, nor could he imagine that he would recover. Believing that his "time had come," he was convinced that he would never return to even a semblance of his former self.

Unable to grieve this loss of control over his life effectively, Carl Nunez focused solely on the negative aspects of his illness, and the depressive feelings of his grief reaction became so entrenched that a profound depression resulted. In an effort to prove to himself that he still ran his own life, Mr. Nunez signed himself out of the hospital against medical advice. Despite protests from the medical staff, who were concerned that his depression would deepen and that he might even attempt suicide, Mr. Nunez chose to leave "this place where they try to tell me how to live, what to eat, when to sleep, and what to do." In terms of the grief process, this was a regression to the first stage—denial—and a dramatic reflection of his inability to resolve his conflicting feelings about the loss of health. When he left the hospital, he was physically stable but significantly impaired psychologically.

As Carl Nunez's case dramatically illustrates, the depressive response to illness can seriously interfere with comprehensive medical care. Depression can induce a sense of hopelessness and worthlessness in which the sufferer no longer cares about regaining his or her health. Emotional withdrawal often results in self-neglect, such as rejecting a prescribed treatment regimen, which ultimately promotes physical decline. A stroke victim, for example, may refuse physical therapy, thereby aggravating the effects of muscle disuse. An individual's ability to rally against physical illness may be so seriously compromised that he or she essentially abandons the will to live—and dies. This has been described as the given-up/giving-up syndrome by George Engel, an internationally renowned psychiatrist most noted for his scholarship in psychosomatic medicine. There is also accumulating evidence that depression diminishes one's immune response against infection, and possibly against tumor growth.

A depressive response to illness can also impede accurate diagnosis. As we have seen, depression alters the body's normal functioning, producing symptoms that can confuse the diagnostic picture. Unless the depression is recognized as such, the symptoms may be incorrectly attributed to disease. A common example of this is seen in the elderly patient who responds to illness with depression. Forgetfulness, impaired concentration, and poor self-care are often interpreted as signs of senile dementia. However, they are also symptoms of a dementialike syndrome that may be caused by depression. In addition, by not recognizing the signs and symptoms of depression, the medically ill patient may fail to appreciate his or her clinical improvement. If this causes the patient to reject recommended treatment, it may actually aggravate physical distress.

Finally, depression can progress in severity to the degree

that it becomes a greater health threat than the physical illness and necessitates psychiatric treatment. Under these circumstances, the physician's ability to help the patient recover is gravely limited, especially when the patient's outlook on life is captured by Carl Nunez's resigned question "What's the use?"

9

The Dependency Response

Some people regress when subjected to excessive stress. They revert to behaviors characteristic of earlier developmental stages. Regression temporarily renders the individual more dependent; but it also permits an emotional retrenchment that can alleviate anxiety and enhance psychological strength. In this manner, regression serves both an adaptive and a defensive purpose. A person's return to familiar behavior provides a kind of emotional comfort— an escape from the apprehension and uncertainties that are part of adulthood. Uncharacteristic immature behavior usually elicits the attention and support the person requires from those close to him or her. This kind of regressed behavior is analogous to a needy child's request for parental help. Regression, characterized by self-absorption and some degree of irresponsibility, serves as an emotional time-out when coping with the current stresses in life becomes too difficult.

Regression is an integral part of illness, since disease forces us to become more dependent on those around us. When we feel badly, we enjoy being cared for, wanting to be tended to and then left alone. After recovery, we return to our previous level of physical and mental well-being. When hospitalization is required, regression becomes even more pronounced. Many people regard hospitalization as a form of incarceration. Although they may appreciate the therapeutic purpose of their confinement, the loss of autonomy leaves them feeling helpless and inadequate—almost completely overtaken by their caretakers.

It is not surprising that many patients feel that they have little or no control over themselves. As the self-perception of being small, helpless individuals increases, they invest caretakers with increasing amounts of omnipotence. This regressive experience is often demoralizing and frightening, but it's the price patients pay for the expectation of specific rewards. They expect expert attention from a medical community that provides a thorough workup, a correct diagnosis, and careful explanations, empathic treatment, and recovery. Unconsciously, they think that if they behave like obedient children, they should also reap considerable benefit—namely, good health—from those who are perceived as benign parental figures.

The Sick Role

The sociologist Talcott Parsons's discussion of *the sick role* offers a framework for looking at how illness can affect a person's social and psychological functioning. Parsons identified four distinct phases of the sick role, the first of which is "exemption from normal social role responsibilities." The permissible degree of exemption is determined by the nature and severity of the illness and is legitimized by a physician's dispensation. The next aspect of the sick role is the recognition by both patient and health care providers that a recovery cannot be effected simply by willing it. At this stage, there is an increasing dependency on the caretakers. The final two stages of the sick role are the most relevant for an understanding of the dependency response to illness. In the third phase, the patient recognizes the undesirability of ill health and begins to strive for wellness. This is accomplished in the final stage, when the ailing individual seeks help from and cooperates with healers in the recovery process. At this point, medical treatment becomes a collaborative effort—what Parsons called a "common task."

Maintaining a balance between the adaptive and the defensive aspects of regression serves to maximize chances for successful treatment. In the progression toward wellness, regression becomes less and less desirable; it may even become an impediment to regaining functioning. As recovery progresses, the patient comes to rely less on health care personnel and more on his or her own abilities to be independent. Should the patient resist this evolution, regression becomes excessive, either in degree or in duration. Then dependency makes it impossible to reassume previous responsibilities.

Case Studies: Sheldon May and Stewart Harrington

Sheldon May had a stroke at age sixty-eight. When he was hospitalized during the acute phase, virtually all he was capable of doing was to wait passively and see if he would survive the catastrophe. Once his condition stabilized and he became aware of the extent of his impairment (slurred speech and slight stiffness on one side of his body), the major responsibility for further successful treatment fell on his shoulders. He was sent to rehabilitative personnel who taught him to live as effectively as possible with his impairment. At the same time, Sheldon learned how to do things for himself. In physical therapy, he continually challenged himself to see how many more steps he could take, and he asked for extra sessions with a speech therapist to work on returning his speech to normal. Mr. May progressed through the stages of the sick role in the anticipated manner. He and his caregivers felt confident about his ability to make a good recovery and continue to live a reasonably independent life.

Stewart Harrington, on the other hand, who was also

sixty-eight years old, did not accommodate as effectively to his stroke. He often spoke of his inability to control the weakness in his right side and demanded to be moved in a wheelchair, rather than relearning how to walk. This increased the risk of muscle atrophy and therefore enhanced debility. He repeatedly asked to see his doctor and the various therapists who were treating him. Rather than developing his independence by learning how to function with his disabilities, he abdicated responsibility for his care—and his progress—by continually turning to others for help. Mr. Harrington reaped some rewards by remaining dependent, most likely the alleviation of anxiety through external support. He clearly preferred those rewards to the satisfaction of self-realized achievement.

This kind of helpless behavior can seriously disrupt the collaborative aspect of the physician-patient relationship; the physician becomes frustrated with his or her increasing responsibilities for the patient's welfare, while the patient pays the insidious price of progressive helplessness.

Patients like Stewart Harrington only partly fulfill the criteria of the sick role. They gladly seek and accept the attention of their caretakers, who, by legitimizing their illness, grant exemptions from society's rules and responsibilities. However, they do not truly cooperate in their treatment, because they do not really wish to get well. With either conscious or unconscious behavior, these patients resist and undermine the best efforts of their caretakers. All such patients impede their own progress, at the same time frustrating their caretakers. A struggle often evolves between the patient who is committed to remaining ill and the physician whose mission it is to see the patient recover. The patient usually wins the battle, and suffers the consequences, which range from functioning at a lower level than that warranted by the illness to assuming the role of "professional patient." This type of person, obsessed with his or her state of health, is forever discovering new symptoms and fearing the onset of new ailments. Consequently, he or she submits to extensive diagnostic workups and therapeutic regimens in order to manage what is frequently an easily treatable (and sometimes even nonexistent) problem. Thus passivity, worry, and neediness ultimately make it impossible to enjoy life's pleasures.

Case Study: Elizabeth Werner

Elizabeth Werner, a seventy-two-year-old, was admitted to the mental health unit of a hospital for evaluation of her progressively impaired functioning over the preceding five years following open-heart surgery. Numerous diagnostic tests failed to demonstrate any physical cause for her decline, and her internist suspected a psychiatric disorder.

At the time of her admission, she had been neglecting all but the most basic activities of daily life. She professed a strong desire to resume her previously responsible routine but said that it was "beyond hope to be the way I was before they operated on me." Her surgery took place three years after a heart attack. Ms. Werner was unable to articulate exactly how the surgery produced her prolonged debility, especially in light of the fact that it significantly reduced her symptoms. She did, however, communicate her inability to do anything but read and do crossword puzzles.

Throughout her life, Elizabeth Werner was a vigorous, responsible woman who took great pride in her abilities and achievements as a wife and mother. Although her life was not without difficulty, including the rearing of a daughter with diabetes, she had few complaints. She dealt with adversity philosophically, regarding it as unavoidable. Ms. Werner's gradual but persistent decline began shortly after her open-heart surgery.

Over time, she became completely dependent on her husband and was terrified of losing him. She let herself become housebound, and her friends gradually drifted away. She was very self-conscious about the effect of her extreme dependence on her family and was emotionally agitated about her situation. Mounting physical complaints required several rehospitalizations, though none of the tests showed any significant findings. She consulted a psychiatrist, who believed her behavior was due to an underlying depression. He prescribed a course of antidepressants, but this failed to relieve her symptoms.

Ms. Werner felt the psychiatrist had not helped her at all, despite twice-weekly meetings and the use of various medications for more than a year. In fact, she wasn't even certain what the psychiatrist expected from the current hospitalization. She also felt that she didn't "fit in" at this hospital because, as she stated, "I'm just like a zombie. I'm always too tired."

Given her past medical history—two previous operations that went smoothly and from which she recovered quickly—it was unclear exactly why Ms. Werner regressed so profoundly after her cardiac surgery. There are several possible explanations for this. First, both of her parents died in their seventies of cardiovascular disease, a family history that might have sensitized Ms. Werner to the impact of heart disease late in life. Another possible explanation has to do with her cardiac operation. Anticipating routine bypass surgery, she awoke from anesthesia to learn of an unplanned repair of an aneurysm (a swelling) of the heart wall. This "surprise" could have increased her uncertainty about her condition in general, causing a pathologic vigilance that was her attempt to prevent any further surprises. A third possibility is that Ms. Werner's behavior was an unconscious expression of anger. Throughout her life, she was the family caretaker. Her persistent helplessness could be a way of demanding the attention and support she felt she deserved.

The latter explanation seemed the most plausible. Unconscious dependency had prevented Ms. Werner from continuing her previous self-sufficient existence. She expressed concern about the detrimental effects of her current reliance on her family. Nevertheless, she continued her demands for support by becoming increasingly helpless and isolated. Seemingly at the mercy of those around her, she asserted control over them by her passivity. Her inability to do anything for herself was a loud demand to be cared for, and her family, motivated by a combination of concern and guilt, complied. In actuality, Ms. Werner's debility provided her with great power over those close to her.

Ambivalent about her helplessness, Ms. Werner was unable to comprehend the part of her that no longer wanted to function as she used to. Consequently, she could not overtly request support from her loved ones because to do so would reverse established family roles. At the same time, her illness permitted her to silently—and successfully—solicit the assistance she craved. This secondary gain is an integral part of the dependency response. Unfortunately, the benefits that are realized through illness are usually offset by their great emotional cost. In Ms. Werner's case, the price was significant: in addition to transforming her into a marginally functional woman isolated from her friends, her response alienated her children and medical caretakers and stressed her husband to the breaking point. Furthermore, the luxury derived from her total dependence on her husband—alleviation of all responsibilities—was accompanied by an ever-present terror that something would happen to him. Ms. Werner's pathologic dependency made her childlike and so helpless that it is difficult to imagine her ever having functioned in a self-reliant fashion—or ever doing so again.

A dependency response is not always obvious. Sometimes it is disguised behind a false bravado. In such a case, the patient never openly declares his or her extreme wishes for dependency, either because of an unconscious desire for self-deception about these regressive needs, or because of a conscious, more deliberate manipulative intent. Regardless of motivation, concealing the need for excessive nurturing confuses caretakers: the patient overtly declares his or her independence while behaving in a regressive manner. Eventually, the therapeutic relationship is disrupted by a struggle between the patient, who wishes to remain ill (even if this is not admitted), and caretakers, who are committed to making the patient well. This shadowy battle, while appearing completely different from the warfare between Ms. Werner and her doctors, holds the same consequences for the patient: psychological and physical regression that limits independent functioning.

Case Study: Bruce Youngman

The case of Bruce Youngman illustrates this second type of dependency response. Mr. Youngman is a forty-two-year-old married man with three children, who are between the ages of ten and fifteen. A carpenter by trade, he runs his own business. He was in good health until he was involved in a car accident; eighteen months later he ventured into the hospital. Although the accident left him bruised and shaken, he had no obvious injuries and returned to work the same afternoon. Several days later he was awakened in the middle of the night by severe abdominal pain. Despite numerous visits to different physicians and many medical interventions, the pain persisted unabated since that time, and, according to Mr. Youngman, it ruined his life.

Mr. Youngman underwent exploratory surgery and claimed the doctors removed the entire pancreas, the spleen, and the gallbladder. But he had exaggerated the extent of his operation—only part of his pancreas had been surgically removed. He purposely distorted his history, as opposed to misperceiving what he had been told of his illness.

Mr. Youngman's pain persisted for months. He again consulted the surgeon, who, he claimed, told him he had a chronic pancreatitis that there was no cure for and that would be a source of pain for the rest of his life. The doctor suggested that he visit the pain clinic at the hospital, where he would be equipped with an electronic device used to help alleviate chronic pain. The doctor also told him that if the electric stimulation didn't work, he could have a nerve block. Mr. Youngman was currently existing on heavy doses of narcotics because he said he couldn't function without them. However, he was building up a tolerance to the drugs. He also stated: "Because I can no longer function with the pain, my business is standing still."

Mr. Youngman projected an image of determined response to adversity. He attempted to communicate a supposed ability to be assertive and strong in the face of a purported "hellish" twenty-four-hour-a-day pain. The real feelings behind his bravado surfaced, however, during an incident where an intern inserted an intravenous catheter and Mr. Youngman howled with pain. He insisted on having a nurse give him a shot for the pain immediately. Afterward, he dwelled on the horrible, distracting pain he was experiencing from his condition and went so far as to offer an award of $10,000 to anyone within a group of visiting medical students who could take his pain away. These actions communicated the underlying dependency that played a significant role in his chronic pain.

Mr. Youngman's illness response was characterized by an overriding reliance on others to make him well. He opted to become a passive participant in his treatment because of an inability to cope with his illness. He abdicated to one of his physicians complete control over decisions such as discharge from the hospital and hinted at finding a psychiatrist who could tell him what to do. Despite his professed desire to return to work, his opposition to independent functioning became increasingly obvious. He claimed to be out of shape, and feared that that would prevent him from working effectively for a little while, reflecting both a concern and a wish. He feared chronic debilitation; but at the same time, he desired the helplessness in which he had luxuriated for eighteen months. Not only did his regression excuse him from work, it also prompted sympathy and nurturance from family, friends, and a large number of physicians.

It was impossible to get a clear picture of Bruce Youngman's illness dynamics because of his guardedness. However, the limited information he did share enabled the therapist to form a hypothesis: Mr. Youngman's father was a compulsive worker who "worked himself into a bad heart" and then a fatal heart attack. His mother died grieving her husband. Perhaps Mr. Youngman believed that hard work and continued health were incompatible; not only did the patient suffer, but so did the patient's loved ones. In response to his father's maladaptive illness response—excessive denial—Mr. Youngman may have responded to ill health in exactly the opposite manner. He became helpless and forced himself to contain his competitive urges, fearing they might get out of control and drive him inexorably to debility and death. Paradoxically, in his effort to stay healthy, he was actually contributing to his decline in health.

Bruce Youngman's case vividly illustrates how important it is for physicians to recognize a patient's disguised dependency as early in the treatment as possible. By misinterpreting false bravado as gutsy determination, by reading passivity as motivation, the physician may overestimate the patient's desire and willingness to work collaboratively to get well. This can lead to unrealistic expectations, such as discharging a postoperative patient ahead of the usual timetable owing to the physician's (incorrect) perception that the patient is ready for release. The person who is secretly dependent often feels overwhelmed by this aggressive treatment approach and regresses to an even greater degree. The struggle that ensues—the physician becomes increasingly dedicated to helping a patient who secretly wishes to remain ill—has harmful consequences. The physician may view persisting symptoms as glaring examples of professional inadequacy, causing him or her to feel helpless and frustrated in attempting to cure the patient. Should these feelings continue, the physician might eventually be angrily driven to acting them out, ordering numerous diagnostic tests, unnecessary therapeutic procedures, or medications. Bruce Youngman's drug dependence was certainly encouraged by his physicians' repeated attempts to silence complaints of pain by pharmacologic means. The anger component of a patient's dependency response—his or her demand to be made well—is matched by the angry caretakers' control over the patient. The dangerous competition that results is one that occurs frequently when a physician is treating someone who attempts to hide his or her extreme dependency.

The dependency response to illness occurs whenever a person believes that the sick role, as described by Parsons, brings more rewards than the return to health. That circumstance undermines the motivation to work collaboratively with caretakers. Instead, the person remains in an excessively regressed state, choosing the attention and nurturance of caretakers over the return to autonomous functioning.

10

Illness and the Family

Illness is not simply an individual experience. When a person becomes ill, the emotional balance of the entire family unit is disrupted. The degree of disruption is influenced by such factors as which family member is sick, what the prognosis is, what care will be necessary, the expected duration of the acute episode, whether hospitalization is required, and who will care for the patient later.

Whatever the individual circumstances of a family, one thing is certain: each family member has intense and varied feelings about the illness of one of its members. In addition, the family *as a unit* will respond in a characteristic way, and that way will be different for every family. Families that can express the feelings precipitated by the illness, and at the same time retain their ability to do the kind of rational problem solving necessary in times of crisis, are best equipped to deal with this kind of difficult situation.

Case Study: Marsha Jacobson

Marsha Jacobson is a forty-two-year-old who has three children, ages eight, twelve, and fifteen, and who works part-time as a legal secretary. Her husband, Phil, owns his own consulting business, which requires him to travel approximately three days every month.

One day Ms. Jacobson developed severe, intermittent stomach pain accompanied by nausea. Preliminary findings after a medical history, physical, and initial blood tests suggested that Ms. Jacobson had gallbladder disease. The definitive X-ray tests were scheduled for two weeks later.

Ms. Jacobson and her husband worried about the outcome of the tests, and although they didn't discuss it, each was concerned about the improbable—but possible—diagnosis of cancer. Their way of dealing with their concerns was to spend more time together, trying to be mutually reassuring and supportive. During the same period, two of their children became uncharacteristically difficult. The eight-year-old complained twice of a stomachache and refused to go to school one day. The twelve-year-old complained that his parents weren't offering their usual help with homework assignments.

When the subsequent tests were finally done, they confirmed the physician's original suspicion: Ms. Jacobson had multiple gallstones that caused periodic inflammation of her gallbladder. The Jacobsons greeted this news with concern and relief. Knowing the diagnosis allowed the Jacobsons to pull the family together and get back to its old routines. Much of the tension evaporated that had been present in the household while Ms. Jacobson's medical condition was being evaluated.

After she was diagnosed, Ms. Jacobson had some decisions to make concerning her treatment options. The illness could be treated medically, that is, with a controlled diet and medications she could take when the pain and nausea flared up. Or she could choose to have her gallbladder surgically removed. She decided to have surgery.

Ms. Jacobson had to make a decision concerning the timing of the operation. Many family considerations came into play. Her own work schedule was flexible and could easily accommodate the period of hospitalization and convalescence. Her husband had some previously scheduled out-of-town business commitments that he wanted to keep. It was also necessary to find someone to take care of the children. Ms. Jacobson's older sister, who lived in another city, agreed to come and spend one or two weeks to run the house, look after the children, and nurse Ms. Jacobson while she recuperated at home. Mr. Jacobson and his wife told the children about her surgery and informed them that activities would be somewhat curtailed during her hospitalization and period of recuperation. He made two suggestions: that they ask friends to help out, and that they temporarily select only those activities that were most important to them. In this way, the children were also prepared for the reality of their mother's hospitalization and convalescence and were able to be less demanding than usual in order to help out.

The surgery took place on schedule and went well. After a brief hospital stay, Ms. Jacobson was released and returned home. Although her physicians were satisfied with her progress, she was in considerably more pain than she had anticipated. She disliked the pain medication her physician had prescribed, complaining that it made her feel "too groggy," but she continued taking it because of her discomfort. During her first postoperative week, she was surprised at how tired she felt. When her husband tried to reassure her, she initially rejected his encouragement as patronizing but soon recognized that he was trying to comfort her. Ms. Jacobson had some other concerns at this time: she felt guilty about the amount of time her husband was spending away from his office, and she was also worried about the cost of her treatment and whether her husband would be able to take care of the family's financial matters during her convalescence.

During the next couple of weeks Ms. Jacobson started to feel better. She sent her sister home, thanking her for her assistance. Next she resumed her role in her children's daily routine, even attending a school play put on by her eight-year-old's class. She began planning her return to work. Eventually, she was back to her normal routine. At first, her family hovered around her, continually warning her "not to overdo it." While she was initially pleased by the attention and concern her family was showing, she began to get annoyed by their anxiety and politely told them that she was feeling well and they shouldn't worry. When her husband refused to make love because it was so soon after her operation, she became angry with him because she felt fine.

Follow-up visits with her surgeon confirmed that she was doing as well as she thought. Her husband remarked that he was grateful that she was feeling better, and he hoped this was "the end" of her problems. Subsequently, both of them admitted that although they believed she was cured, they still had minor worries that this might not have been the definitive treatment, and that she might eventually have complications from the surgery. They agreed that they would feel more secure with her cure if she remained without symptoms for several months to come. Fortunately, as the following years proved, she was indeed cured of her illness.

The Family Process Response to Illness

Although a family is an aggregate of individuals, it is also a distinctive unit that responds to life circumstances in characteristic ways. When family members come together, they generate predictable patterns of interaction under normal circumstances and under stressful situations such as illness in a relative. These characteristic patterns are known as *family process responses*. They are like chemical reactions that result when different materials are combined: when separate, the ingredients exhibit their unique properties; when mixed together, they can form an entirely new substance with different properties.

The family process response to illness represents how a family handles its emotional issues, in other words, how the illness becomes integrated into the family's basic pattern of experiencing and coping with stress. The Jacobson family exhibited a normal family process response to illness. Everyone experienced some degree of anxiety, physical and emotional strain, and hardship owing to Ms. Jacobson's gallbladder disease. However, the individual family members offered support and understanding to one another, which ultimately benefited everyone. As their case illustrates, the family process response involves emotional, cognitive, and interpersonal issues.

When illness strikes a family member, the unit undergoes an *emotional readjustment* similar to the grief process discussed earlier (see Chapter 3). Many feelings—both positive and negative—are experienced, expressed, and ultimately resolved. This occurs simultaneously on two levels: the individual family members' personal response to the illness, and the collective emotional response of the family as a unit. All family members, not just the patient, must gain a perspective on the illness of a loved one in order to place the episode—whether long- or short-term—into the family's collective experience and history.

On the *cognitive level*, the family becomes educated about all the aspects of the disease in question. They learn the symptoms, the treatment, the complications, and the prognosis. Such knowledge grants family members a degree of mastery over the situation. Knowledge—particularly when all family members have the same knowledge—enables them to plan together. They can divide responsibilities, help select treatments, make arrangements for care. They know what must be done to assist the patient in combating the illness. Without this shield of knowledge, the family can easily become ruled by emotions, leaving each family member unable to deal effectively with stress and more susceptible to nonproductive responses.

On an *interpersonal level*, adjustments to interactions must be made by healthy family members with one another, with medical personnel, and with the patient. The interpersonal adjustments, both within and outside the family, are closely tied to the family's emotional responses. The illness of a single family member is prone to change the usual style of interpersonal relationships among all family members. An individual whose usual response to stress is to become controlling, or passive, or withdrawn, may become even more so; the family accommodates to these exaggerated responses by making changes in its internal interactions.

When illness strikes, the family process reaction reflects the extreme interdependence of family members. In Marsha Jacobson's case, the patient's emotional response to disease affected the family's emotional response to the disease, which, in turn, affected her reaction, and there was a constant interplay between these two forces. This ongoing process can be either beneficial or detrimental, depending on whether it helps the patient and family to grieve effectively the patient's loss of health and its subsequent effects on the family. As a result, the family process reaction influences the course of an illness, as well as the stability and functioning of the family unit.

The family process reaction consists of a number of distinct phases: (1) recognizing that someone is ill; (2) determining what is wrong; (3) obtaining the necessary treatment; and (4) reestablishing a normal equilibrium following treatment, which may require making permanent changes in the family roles and the operation of the family. This four-stage response closely parallels the grief response experienced by an individual who becomes ill.

Phase I: Onset of Illness

During this initial phase, the meaning of an illness is incorporated into a family system. This is often a subtle process, the impact of which increases over time. Consider the case of Douglas Epstein, age sixty-two. A heavy smoker for more than forty years, Mr. Epstein noticed a decrease in his energy level over the past few months. This began to affect his—and his family's—behavior. He and his wife, Cynthia, canceled a vacation. They began to curtail their social activities. Their sex life suffered. As they altered their life-style to accommodate Doug's changed physical condition, both he and Cynthia experienced losses. Others experienced these losses, as well: children and other family members, friends, even business acquaintances. This marked the beginning of a sequence of changes that evolves in any family that can no longer function in its customary manner.

At some point, the person or someone close to him or her begins to consciously associate some of the physical symptoms with changes in behavior. This association raises some questions and worries, most notably the question of what might be wrong. In Doug Epstein's case, it was his boss—also a social acquaintance—who noticed that the Epsteins had canceled a number of social engagements over the past few months, and that Mr. Epstein did not have any enthusiasm for his job. His boss suggested that he get a checkup, and his wife seconded the idea. He was diagnosed with emphysema.

Once Mr. Epstein realized that there was something physically wrong with him, he began to worry about Cynthia: whether she would be able to contend with his illness, whether she would be widowed at an early age. Cynthia Epstein was naturally concerned about her husband's health, and she was also worried about the financial consequences of his illness. The members of the family now began to realize that the life of the patient, and in turn their day-to-day lives, might be altered by his illness.

The pattern just described can be linked to a relatively slow onset of illness. In such a situation, there are few immediate *concrete* effects on the patient and his or her family. They may spend time, as the Epsteins did, speculating about the future and in a state of uncertainty about what will occur. They may wonder about the diagnosis and the consequences of treatment. Will surgery cause disfigurement, or will chemotherapy be debilitating? How will the patient respond to that? How will the family respond? How will the family react to the patient's response?

On the other hand, when an illness comes on suddenly—and seriously—there is a much more pronounced degree of disruption and disorganization in the family. Two examples of sudden onset are the heart attack in a seemingly healthy individual and the serious accident. In such cases, the family is given little, if any, time to attend to emotional adjustment, or to practical matters, such as arranging for the children's transportation to school during a parent's hospitalization, seeking medical advice, and making an educated decision concerning treatment. Many decisions must be made immediately, and the family tends to feel passive, or that the fate of their loved one is out of their control.

In a very real sense, the way the illness declares itself at the time of onset sets in motion a particular family response. Moreover, this initial phase may suggest how the family will react to the illness over its course, as it progresses.

Phase II: Impact

This phase is less speculative, because the illness is defined in a more reality-based fashion than before. The patient and family are informed of the actual diagnosis and of the planned treatment and prognosis. Speculation gives way to real knowledge, and the family can now begin to work through the emotions precipitated by that knowledge.

During this stage, the patient usually undergoes diagnostic procedures. At best, these are anxiety provoking, for the patient awaits test results and can only hope that they will not suggest the diagnosis of a serious or terminal ailment. At worst, diagnostic procedures send patients, and often family members, on a frightening and painful journey. The patient must go to strange places for specialized procedures, be subjected to uncomfortable and embarrassing procedures, and feel completely depersonalized as he or she is probed and examined by complete strangers.

The patient may feel a distinct lack of control over the situation, relying on strangers to determine whether the illness is curable or incurable, painful or not. The entire procedure can be tiring, humiliating, painful, expensive, and thoroughly disruptive to one's daily routine.

The response of each family during this period varies. One may be encouraging and reassuring; another, discouraging; a third, resentful of demands on their time and finances and of the patient's complaints. Furthermore, this diagnostic period seriously involves the family in the patient's illness. It may be only on an emotional level, as they begin to contemplate what will eventually be discovered in the diagnostic workup. Or it may be more active involvement, as when a family member accompanies the patient to tests and procedures or spends a great deal of time listening to the patient express his or her concerns.

Another aspect of the impact phase is *labeling*. After the diagnostic workup, the patient and family are told the specifics of what is wrong. They are given a name for the illness, and they are told what the illness implies. Now begins a period of education. Patient and family ask medical personnel their many questions: What exactly is this illness? What are the types of treatment for it: medication, surgery, radiation, chemotherapy? Will there be any changes in diet or life-style? Is it an acute disease that goes away or a chronic disease that recurs or just gets progressively worse? What is the ultimate prognosis? Can the patient return to normal functioning? Will the patient's functioning be partially compromised? Or will the patient be completely unable to function?

In addition, the process of self-education begins during this phase. Patient and family read books or articles about the illness, ask friends or colleagues about their own experiences, and get in contact with relevant groups, such as the American Heart Association.

During this phase, health care personnel can generally perceive how the family will eventually respond to the patient's illness. Once the problem is diagnosed and *labeled*, caregivers usually know what the course and prognosis will be, and they communicate this information to the family. At this point, a collective grieving process starts, wherein the patient and other family members try to digest the news of the illness and work through their associated emotions, including denial, anger, and ultimately acceptance. These emotional responses will be reflected in their behavior toward the patient and can have a major impact on whether the patient gets what he or she needs in terms of both treatment and his or her general welfare.

There are typically two types of family responses to illness at this stage. In one scenario, the family pulls together. They understand what is happening and recognize the need for mutual support in order to attend to the main task at hand: caring for the sick family member and maintaining optimal family functioning at the same time. As we saw in the case of Marsha Jacobson, there are often negative or difficult feelings associated with this adaptive period. One of the feelings family members experience at this time is *guilt*. The patient's loved ones might say things like, "I should have been able to prevent her from getting sick. I should have watched her diet more closely." Sometimes family members feel *anger*—at the patient for disrupting family routines or at the doctors for a variety of reasons including their role as bearers of bad news. Another common—and understandable—reaction is *depression*. These negative feelings—and others the family members might experience—are all within the bounds of normal behavior. In a normal family situation, both the positive and the negative feelings occur, and as these feelings are worked through, members derive a sense of perspective about what is happening. It is important that, like the patient, the other family members have the opportunity to ventilate their negative feelings so that they also can come to terms with the situation and proceed with the task at hand, which is caring for the sick person.

In the second scenario, we see the beginnings of several types of pathological, or destructive, family responses to the illness of one of its members. They often begin as low-level events with no particular intensity. Some of the patterns seen include: a helplessness and hopelessness that pervades the family; quarrels among family members or with medical personnel; or a minimization—or even complete denial—of what the family has been told throughout the diagnosis and labeling period.

There is something else that usually occurs during this phase, something that takes place outside the family but that has a significant impact within the family unit. Friends and colleagues often make well-intentioned attempts to reassure the patient or other family members after the diagnosis is known. They may try to accentuate the positive or try in other ways to cheer everyone up. Support from outsiders is desirable and can often yield positive effects. However, they must show a certain amount of sensitivity. At this stage, it is all too easy for these attempts at buoying the patient and the family to cause problems. The messages they are receiving from nonmedical personnel may distort or contradict everything they have been told up to this point. This can confuse, or even subvert, the family's normal adaptation to the patient's illness. Most often, this happens when the patient or individual family members are seduced by the comforting words of friends and acquaintances into not considering some of the possibly dire consequences of a diagnosed illness. The input of friends may actually support a pathological response within the family—denial, for example—which ultimately has a detrimental result for both patient and family.

Phase III: Treatment

In this phase of major therapeutic effort, there is ample opportunity for the family to work together on the specific task at hand: namely, helping the patient get better. Often, family members are called upon to provide *real, tangible support*; to *do things* for the patient that he or she is unable to do. For example, someone with a leg in a cast may need

family members to help with bathing; and someone recuperating in bed might need someone to do the grocery
shopping and prepare meals. The family tends to the needs
of the patient, often assuming both minor and major responsibilities such as performing chores around the house
and offering financial support while the patient cannot
work.

Family members can also provide *psychological support*
to the patient. Sometimes, simply being present and available communicates to the patient that he or she needn't
worry about being taken care of. Since people who are sick
often fear that they won't be able to take care of themselves, that reassurance can be a valuable elixir. The family can also offer suggestions to the patient, such as gently
encouraging more physical activity, and urging the patient
to take a painkiller or sleeping pill when it appears that
it would be helpful but he or she is resisting. An important
role the family can play is in helping the patient acknowledge and ventilate his or her emotions about the illness.
Family members can share their own feelings and in this
way encourage the patient to do the same. This can help
significantly by setting in motion the normal grieving process that the patient must experience.

As the patient's condition improves or stabilizies, the
family's role begins to change. Now they must help the
patient become more autonomous, assigning increasing
responsibility and encouraging the resumption of normal
activities and life-style. This comes about either as a result
of direct and purposeful discussions among the family
members or through a general, unstated acknowledgment
that the patient is better and can get back to the usual
routine. For example, family members who have been
pitching in may deem that the patient is now ready to
resume driving and no longer needs to be chauffeured
around.

Sometimes, one or more family members, for reasons
of their own, do not encourage the patient back from the
increased dependency brought on by ill health. Instead,
they do things that infantilize the patient and keep him

or her in a dependent role. Some patients succumb to such infantilization by family members, either because they are not physically or emotionally strong enough to fight it, or because they willingly welcome it. Whatever the motivation, this passive response to illness often inhibits the return to healthy functioning.

During the treatment phase it is normal for family members' reactions to vary over time. They may be hypervigilant, closely observing the patient for the slightest nuances of change, even if treatment has just begun. Or they may be periodically angry or depressed or helpless. These feelings—and the shifting between them—is as much a function of their real observations of the patient as it is of their own feelings about the family member's illness.

There is much less uncertainty during this phase than during the two preceding ones. The problem has already been isolated and diagnosed; therapy has already been instituted; and markers for the effectiveness of treatment, in the form of certain symptoms or degree of functioning, have been identified. The availability of more objective criteria during this phase removes some of the uncertainty of earlier phases, which in turn may help both patient and family come to terms with the illness, its treatment, and prognosis.

The degree of both short-term and longer-term disruption generally becomes more evident during this treatment phase. Several weeks of treatment or convalescence give the family some sense of what to expect in terms of recovery: whether the paralysis or speech loss of the stroke patient improves: whether the patient who suffered a heart attack has any angina or congestive heart failure; or how well the patient's medications seem to be working. They get a notion of how much exertion the patient will be able to tolerate and begin to understand what to expect in terms of a return to normal routine. During this phase, family members also get a sense of the financial consequences of illness: how much the medical bills are and what their insurance will cover; whether the patient will be able to return to work. In addition, any changes to the basic patterns of relationship within the family start to become evident at this point. Will the prior primary wage earner now become the dependent spouse? Will one child be receiving considerably more attention than before, and, consequently, will the parents or siblings be receiving less from one another? There is tremendous opportunity during the treatment phase for family patterns to be disrupted. This disruption can have serious consequences for the patient's recovery as well as for the emotional well-being of other family members.

Phase IV: Adjustment to Treatment Outcome

This phase is generally of longer duration than the treatment phase and is divided into an early and late period. It is analogous to the resolution, or acceptance, phase of normal grief experienced by the patient, but now all the family members are involved. The net result at the end of this stage is that the family as a unit, and as individuals, resolve the emotions precipitated by the patient's illness.

This phase is affected by the patient's prognosis and the degree of functioning that is ultimately expected. The answers to questions that may have been asked at earlier stages—and were unanswerable then—become clearer. How debilitated will the patient be? How much will he or she be able to do? Will the patient return to his or her usual level of functioning, or will there be any residual deficits? Once the family finds answers to these—and similar—questions, a change occurs. Now there is a shift, often subtle, in the family's perception of the patient from being sick to being recovered.

Of course, this shift is influenced by the kind of illness involved. If the illness is chronic, recovery is transient and may just represent improvement from a single, acute episode; it's only a *relative recovery*. On the other end of the spectrum is the patient who suffers from a single, acute episode of an illness, like appendicitis. Once the patient is healed from the surgery and the convalescence period is over, he or she is totally recovered. The recovery is not relative or conditional.

Labeling the Return to Health

Just as the early stage of illness necessitates a *labeling of the illness*, the final phase requires a *labeling of the return to health*. Family and caregivers all assert that the patient is fully recovered. It is then up to the patient to accept that judgment.

Sometimes this poses a different kind of problem for the patient because of what psychiatrists call *secondary gain*. The term refers to the obvious gratification or benefits that are realized because of an illness, the most usual being the care, attention, and nurturance that the patient receives. As discussed by Parsons (see Chapter 9), the sick role allows a person to solicit succor from family members, friends, health care providers—with little fear that requests for help will be denied. In addition to receiving treatment for physical problems, being sick entitles the person to expect, or even demand, considerable support in getting through the stressful period of illness. This support is a form of emotional nourishment and includes reassurance, sympathy, concern, encouragement, and a variety of other positive emotions. Although these feelings intermittently characterize all relationships, they rarely occur in such concentrated form as when one is ill. Consequently, being labeled healthy carries the price of having to give up this considerable nurturance, which is not always easy to do. As a result, patients sometimes try to "hold on" to their symptoms, exaggerating, even fabricating some complaints in order to perpetuate this secondary gain of an illness.

Being sick also permits the abdication of daily responsibilities, which relates to another aspect of secondary gain. The teenager who sustains a sports injury might actually prefer a prolonged recuperation. Although being laid up means missing some sporting events, it also excuses the teenager from household chores or errands, which is experienced as a "positive" aspect of the injury. Such secondary gain is usually unconscious, an automatic behavior by patients who appreciate that there are some plusses to the illness state. Mr. Youngman (see Chapter 9) provides an excellent example of secondary gain. Because of his chronic pain, he was prescribed excessive amounts of narcotics, which not only made him feel good but simultaneously dulled his emotions about being sick—and gave him the perfect excuse to retreat from business responsibilities. Secondary gain can also be a conscious behavior, such as exaggerating the physical effects of an automobile accident or a work-related injury to reap financial benefits. This is in fact *malingering*, consciously exploiting specific rewards of the sick role.

It is important to remember that illness causes dependency, and most people want to give up that dependency and return to as high a level of functioning as possible. Most families concur with that wish. Hence slowly but steadily the patient makes the adjustment to the outcome of treatment and the family resumes its normal functioning. In some instances, however, a family may actually want to keep the patient more dependent. This response reflects the illness dynamics of individual family members and can result in a family pathologic response to the illness.

The seriousness of the illness affects the labeling of the recovery. In the case of a catastrophic illness (such as a stroke) that leaves the patient severely impaired, "recovery" means the family has to permanently alter its previous patterns of interaction to accommodate the severe debility. This places significant stress on the family as a unit and on its members individually. Families now tend to become aware of the stress they are experiencing. They also realize at this point that there is not going to be a "miracle treatment" that will restore the patient to full health. Instead, they begin to incorporate new tasks or patterns of work into the family unit in order to accommodate to the illness.

It is important to recognize that even when the patient's improvement starts to become apparent, the family may have some negative thoughts. Often, family members become somewhat preoccupied with questions concerning recurrence of the illness, the doctors' accuracy or truthfulness, and the effects of treatment. If the family is too worried about these questions to adequately acknowledge real improvements, this can interfere with their ability to declare the patient "recovered."

Resolution /Acceptance

During the second half of the final stage of the family process reaction, the family comes to an accurate assessment of the illness and its consequences and arrives at a true resolution of the situation.

Most families are willing and happy to return to "normalcy." Even if the patient requires ongoing treatment, the return to whatever semblance of an earlier routine is possible is viewed positively; because of the family's adjustment to illness, the treatment will be incorporated into their regular family routine. Life resumes, and everyone picks up his or her previous role, responsibilities, and functions.

An important step in the return to normalcy is when the family begins to treat the patient as recovered— even if there is some persisting impairment or required treatment such as controlled diet, medications, or even limited activity. The family must make the distinction between illness and health, regardless of whether the patient is limited in some way. Dysfunctional families are the ones that focus solely on the limits imposed by the illness. In these families, the patient is declared forever sick. Neglecting someone's obvious strengths—and concentrating on impairment—can sabotage the patient's best attempts at recovery and permanently hamper functioning.

Why Some Families Respond
Abnormally to Illness

The Family as a Group

A large body of psychiatric literature addresses the process of *group interaction* or *group process*, how individuals relate to one another when more than two people are involved. A group is formed when individuals come together to accomplish a task or a collection of related tasks. It is defined solely in terms of that particular goal and is not considered to be a group unless all members are working collectively toward that end. For example, several strangers waiting for a bus are an aggregate of individuals. If, however, they see a pedestrian get hit by a car and mobilize to provide assistance—tending to injuries, calling for an ambulance, summoning the police—they then become a group, individuals united and, therefore, defined by a common task.

The family is a special type of small group. On the one hand, its members lead distinctive lives, characterized by different responsibilities, stresses, and rewards depending on their age and position in the world. In this regard, every family is merely a collection of individuals who tend to their own lives independent of the input of other members. However, the family's predominant existence is as a group, an intimately connected aggregate of people who constantly interact in order to realize the many, interrelated goals that benefit individuals, as well as the family as a whole. For example, parents invest time and energy to ensure that their children receive a good education: they espouse the pleasure and worth of learning, make scheduled visits to their children's schools, help with homework, and discuss with each other any school problems experienced by their children. Similarly, a busy Saturday requires family members to coordinate schedules so that each of them can run necessary errands or participate in recreational activities.

Groups that operate efficiently and effectively are considered work-oriented, or *work groups.* That is not to say that there is always harmony among these people. Tempers can flare, people may avoid one another or openly refuse to work together, or they may challenge one another. But because the group is a productive unit, its members ultimately rise above their interpersonal difficulties to concentrate on the task at hand.

Whenever a group gets together, it also runs the risk of participating in an *abnormal group process* that impedes—or sometimes prevents entirely—the accomplishment of its defined tasks. In this circumstance, the group does not behave in a rational, intelligent manner and does not focus on its true goals. For a variety of reasons endemic to the psychological makeup of its individual members, and to their interaction with one another, the group behaves as if it had other priorities.

Professionals who work with families and other groups have identified three predominant abnormal group processes: the *fight-flight group,* the *dependency group,* and the *pairing group.* These are psychologically unhealthy interactions whose effects are antithetical to the group's successful functioning. Whenever an abnormal group process is operating, the "purpose" of that group is merely to perpetuate that particular type of interaction. For example, if a family is feeling overwhelmed by the catastrophic illness of a member, it may respond with uncharacteristic inadequacy, abdicating all responsibility for medical care to individuals outside the family, such as health providers and friends. All endeavors to promote the family's responsible functioning will be met with its dedicated attempt to increase its helplessness, such as choosing a leader from within whose actions will reaffirm its dependency.

When abnormal group processes prevail in a family, there is a tacit acknowledgment by its members that these nonproductive interactions are more important than adopting a work orientation and completing a necessary task. Here are descriptions of the circumstances of these situations.

Fight-flight. When members assemble, they ultimately end up fighting and struggling, or they withdraw from one another to avoid conflict. The different factions within the group are contentious and unable to compromise or collaborate on a unified program. This type of abnormal group process is largely due to the group's rejection of introspection or self-study. When pursuit of a common task becomes difficult, the group characteristically resorts to *action* to resolve this situation, a type of behavior that permits immediate expression of the emotions plaguing individual group members. They either engage in direct confrontation or calculated moves designed to avoid that conflict. The classic fight-flight group seeks out a leader who consistently promotes turmoil. Whenever the possibility of reconciliation or consensus decision making arises, the leader guides the group in a manner that effectively negates those opportunities.

Dependency. Another maladaptive coping style is for families to become helpless and dependent. In this circumstance nothing is accomplished because the members—individually and collectively—believe they will never achieve their designated task without the assistance of an omniscient, all-powerful leader. As a result, the family continues to regress in a dedicated attempt to entice someone from within its ranks to assume that role. One of two situations usually occurs: the family may remain mired in its paralysis and never achieve its goal; or someone may emerge as a leader and assume all responsibility for decision making. Although the latter circumstance seems preferable, it often perpetuates collective dependency since the designated leader invariably fails to meet the expectations of a significantly regressed family. This usually results in the emergence of another member who similarly fails in the leadership role. But even if this person succeeds in helping the family accomplish a specific work task, the achievement is effected by charisma, not consensus, a further declaration of the group's helplessness. Immaturity, inadequacy, and insecurity characterize the members of a family when the prevailing group process is abnormal dependency. In this emotional environment, even simple tasks become arduous, if not impossible.

Pairing. The final common maladaptive coping style for families involves the process of pairing, where two people bond and assume leadership of the group. The unconscious belief among family members is that something good will emerge from the union of these individuals, an expectation often contradicted by the reality of the situation. For example, two members may be designated to resolve a long-standing difficulty, such as a financial, legal, or health-related matter, which has been overwhelming, if not destructive, to the family. The assumption is that the mere act of assigning responsibility will magically bring about a resolution of the situation. This comes from an unconscious expectation that the two people united have significantly greater knowledge, power, and ability to solve *any* problem.

There are several drawbacks to this group process. First, it is characterized by unfounded hopeful expectation. This fosters a false sense of security and also focuses the family on speculations of a better future at the expense of intelligently addressing the problems and needs of the present. Second, decisions made by the leadership pair are not necessarily informed ones, since they often ignore potentially useful input of other family members. As a result, when a pair initiates action it may do so out of ignorance, which carries obvious risk. Finally, by limiting the significance of most group members, pairing puts distance between the defined pair and the rest of the family. This environment invariably promotes secrets, because the leadership pair becomes privy to information that it judges best not to share. This is a too common occurrence when a family member becomes terminally ill and the leadership pair incorrectly concludes that it is in everyone's best interest to "act normally." When these types of secrets are eventually revealed, as they always are, they often provoke an outpouring of intense negative emotion. Family mem-

bers are angry that they were excluded from such knowledge—despite the fact that they had willingly abdicated
responsibility to the leadership pair—and sad and resentful that they had been deceiving the patient by per-
petuating an atmosphere of happiness and hope when they
should have been preparing the individual, and themselves, for his or her ultimate demise.

The Psychological Health of the Family

Whether or not a family functions as a positive, work-
oriented group is largely determined by the degree of its
basic psychological health. Carl Whitaker, a pioneer in
family therapy, wrote that "the healthy family is one that
continues to grow in spite of whatever trouble comes its
way." Family growth is marked by continued development, individually by its members and collectively as a
unit. The individuals in the family must meet the challenge
of life separate from the family—going off to college or
getting married, for example—while retaining family ties
and remaining supportive of one another. The family must
be able to withstand these stresses, as well as others such
as illness and death.

A healthy family has certain characteristics that enable
it to be flexible in times of stress. Such a family must be
cohesive no matter what stress or conflicts it is undergoing.
All the members share a fundamental belief about that
family: that they will stay together through good and bad
times. There also must be an *openness* about feelings
among family members, a degree of comfort with one another that enables everyone to say what's on their minds.
Individual members should not fear that their emotions
will get out of control if expressed, or that they will have
a devastating effect on other family members. In addition,
individual family members should not feel that others will
retaliate against them for expressing their true feelings.
Independence of the members is encouraged, while the cohesiveness of the family unit is retained. The values of the
healthy family hold that members should go off and do

what's important to them; by so doing, the whole family will in turn be benefited. Finally, the healthy family is *not overly conflicted or extremely controlling of its members.* There are no hidden agendas, no covert forces that affect individual members. Conflicts are openly expressed, and attempts at independence are not sabotaged by other members exerting excessive control over a person's behavior. Families with these characteristics are generally healthier emotionally and usually react to stress—such as the physical illness of a member—in a more healthy and productive manner.

The structural model. This model provides another means for looking at families. It views the family as a single interrelated system with five specific characteristics: (1) the existence of predominant alliances and splits among the members which help establish an equilibrium; (2) a hierarchy of power within the family such as a matriarch or patriarch; (3) clear and firm boundaries between the generations; (4) a tolerance of conflict without using certain individuals as scapegoats; and (5) clear, direct communication among the family members. According to this model, family pathology derives from a change in one or more of these five characteristics. This could be, for example, a shift in predominant alliances, as when one child and one parent become "parents" because the other spouse is not living up to his or her responsibilities. Or the family is thrown into disarray when the usual hierarchy breaks down, as when adolescent children wind up taking care of sickly parents. Major transitions, such as the death of a grandparent or a child coming of age sexually, can also provoke unhealthy psychological functioning in a family.

The family systems model. Murray Bowen devised this theoretical framework for judging the psychological health of a family. This approach evaluates two basic characteristics of the family. First, it assesses the degree of *enmeshment,* or entanglement, present in the family unit. The more the individual members are able to differentiate themselves from one another, the greater the family's ability to cope with significant stress, such as illness in one of its members. Bowen also measures the presence, and effect, of *emotional triangles* in the family. These are three-way subgroups that undermine openness and thereby heighten the level of conflict. Two of the three members of the subgroup are excessively close, which affects the third member but minimizes his or her participation in significant interpersonal interactions. Closeness can be expressed in different ways, including intense love or repetitive conflict. An example of the latter involves a child who usually fights with and irritates one of the parents when they interact. This increases the emotional bond with that parent, albeit in a contentious way, while diluting the degree of intimacy and attachment with the other parent.

The family systems model also argues that pathologic patterns, such as enmeshments and triangles, are repeated over generations and develop into predictable blueprints for the family's behavior. For example, the son of a dependent father may marry an overbearing wife, thereby re-creating the pattern of his parents' marriage.

Families whose usual interactions reflect immature or unhealthy psychological functioning are at particular risk when stressed by illness in a member. Each of the above frameworks demonstrate that openness, flexibility, and established structure within a family help all its members negotiate any period of emotional turmoil. Lacking sufficient psychological health, families are prone to fall into abnormal patterns of group behavior that inhibit or prevent the normal family process response to illness.

Illness Dynamics

Families, like individuals, are subject to illness dynamics. This distinctive network of psychological and social issues can aid or hinder a family's accommodation to sickness in a relative. Internal issues within a family have considerable impact. Some members, for example, readily adjust to illness in themselves or loved ones, which usually helps promote a positive family process response. If, however, other family members have considerable difficulty accepting the effects of illness in a relative, that divergence within the family can cause conflicts that have the potential for producing lasting detrimental effects on the family's emotional life. External issues also contribute to a family's illness dynamics. The availability of health resources, the influence of religion, the presence of social supports, and the effects of cultural mores all have an impact on the family process response.

The specific components of a family's illness dynamics are as varied as those of the individual patient (see Chapter 2). As an illustrative example, consider the stage in the life cycle of a family when illness occurs in one of its members. As a general rule, families are more stable during a particular stage, for example, when children are in primary school or parents are settled in their occupational lives. On the other hand, the changes characteristic of transitional periods are stressful to the family unit. During a pregnancy, or soon after a geographic move, individual members may be too preoccupied to deal optimally with additional stress, such as a sick relative. Alternatively, illness can interfere with the normal transition from one stage to another. Families may reverse decisions concerning planned changes because they feel overly stressed owing to the impact of an illness. Or sickness in a parent may inhibit the developing independence of a late adolescent child who feels too anxious or guilt-ridden to grow increasingly independent of an ailing parent. With chronic illness, the effects on family development can be more profound and long-lasting.

When Children Are Sick

Family members—parents, siblings, close relatives—often find illness in a child particularly distressing. Even a relatively benign condition like an ear infection or a broken bone can cause powerful feelings. People frequently feel helpless in the face of illness; even more so when the sick person is a dependent child.

Many adults find the medical environment a frightening and emotionally debilitating place. It is therefore no surprise that children left to medical personnel, who often cause discomfort, if not outright pain, often become scared and distrustful in that world. They feel abandoned by their parents. They lack the cognitive development to understand what is happening to them—and therefore to help control some of their feelings. For example, it is unlikely that children will be able to conclude intellectually that a biopsy will not be very painful, or that it will be done only once; or that the side effects of a medication will disappear when the medication is stopped; or even that they will feel better in a few days. Furthermore, children don't really understand the reasons for certain procedures that might be uncomfortable or embarrassing.

On the other hand, it's easy to underestimate exactly how much children do understand. Although they may not comprehend medical procedures, they are very sensitive to the emotions of their parents. If the parents are feeling anxious or frightened, the child can sense that, adding to the burden already placed on the latter by illness and treatment. Parents who remain relatively calm and assured serve as good role models for their sick child. Parents should also make an effort to collaborate with the medical staff. The interaction between parents and child should be appropriate and free of the kind of pathological interaction that can interfere with the medical staff's efforts. For example, parents often become excessively nurturing toward a sick child. The benefits of such enhanced support may be outweighed by the significant regression promoted by their efforts, which can interefere with attempts by the medical staff to help the child act more independently. In these circumstances, teaching a juvenile diabetic how to administer insulin, or helping a teenager progress in a rehabilitation program following an accident, becomes that much more difficult for health care providers.

The age of the sick child can have a considerable impact on the family's response. Children five or younger have much greater difficulty tolerating the necessary separations than do older children. Parents therefore will have to invest more time with a younger child than with an older one; for example, taking turns staying overnight with the child in the hospital. Clearly, this has implications for the rest of the family: it is an intrusion on the marital relationship and on the parents' relationship with other children because they are much less available.

Parents will need to take time to educate their child along with providing emotional support. This is particularly true of younger children. It is important that parents be specific with the child, both in terms of the information they present and in ascertaining what the child actually knows and understands. Parents should specifically ask for the child's perceptions about the illness and the treatment, and then, along with medical personnel, try to alter misconceptions and support correct notions.

Siblings, depending on their age and emotional and cognitive maturity, can have a variety of reactions to the illness of a brother or sister. They may fear catching the disease, whether it's possible (as with infectious meningitis) or impossible (as with a broken leg). Sometimes, children feel embarrassed by a sibling's illness, then guilty about their embarrassment. This response is more pronounced when the sibling's appearance is affected: when surgery leads to disfigurement, or when cerebral palsy causes a markedly abnormal gait, or when hair loss follows chemotherapy. Some siblings envy the attention their sick brother or sister receives. They may state so openly or act it out in behaviors designed to get attention for themselves—such as wetting the bed or being disruptive in school. Children can also harbor resentment about the real or imagined burden of responsibility for caring for their sick sibling, either during the current illness or projected long into the future.

A sick sibling can also cause difficulties for the healthy child in the normal quest for independence. Every child has some ambivalence about becoming more independent and moving away from home; it is a natural part of the developmental process. However, concern and guilt about a sick brother or sister and the real need to help out the family may cause healthy siblings to feel more inclined to stay attached to home longer than they would have otherwise.

Parents with a sick child often experience considerable difficulties in their marital relationship. There are a number of reasons for this. One parent may assume more responsibility for the child and consciously or unconsciously become less available to his or her spouse. The spouse who is excluded might begin to resent the partner for spending so much time and paying so much attention to the sick child. He or she might spend increasing amounts of time at work, becoming something of a workaholic in response to the weakened ties of the marriage. Similarly, some people choose to spend more time away from home as a way of escaping from the stress they feel about a child's illness. This also serves to weaken the marital relationship.

Another issue that often arises in the relationship between the parents of a sick child is blame. Parents might consciously or unconsciously accuse each other of causing the child's illness. This might have some basis in reality, as when a child suffers from an accident while being supervised by one of the parents. Or it may be less direct, as when a child develops a hereditary illness, like diabetes, that is present in one of the spouse's families.

How can parents cope with their private feelings about their sick child and handle the strains on their relationship? They are in a better position to do so if they have compatible coping styles. When partners have similar patterns of ego mechanisms and defenses, they usually react to stress in similar ways. Their characteristic responses—which can range from an assertive, take-charge style to a passive, helpless stance—are familiar to both of them. As a result, while they begin adjusting to their child's illness, they go through similar emotional and cognitive processes. This facilitates collaborative work in accommodating to this significant life stress.

A child's illness can provoke a vicious cycle of interpersonal struggles within a family. Both the sick child and the siblings can become more demanding or contentious with the increased stress. Alterations in the usual family routines and interactions can turn a child's world upside down, particularly if he or she is young and inexperienced with life. Parents and medical personnel must make an extra effort to deal sensitively and concretely with both the patient and the healthy siblings in hopes of maintaining some degree of constancy—and therefore security—in the child's life.

Illness is a family affair. When one member becomes sick, it disturbs the family's usual routine. Relatives and members of the immediate social network react to that disturbance, and the patient, in turn, responds to their collective behavior. If the family rallies to help the patient negotiate and adjust to the physical, social, and emotional effects of the illness, the family interaction can be a positive and beneficial experience. Unfortunately, not only are some families ill-equipped to help one of its members contend with illness, they may also actually promote an abnormal illness response in the patient. By focusing exclusively on the physical symptoms, they prevent the open expression of negative feelings, such as anger or depression. Such an atmosphere certainly does not help the patient adapt to the illness. Moreover, it may provide a fertile environment for unhealthy emotional interactions that intermittently occur within the family, even in unstressful times.

11

Negotiating the Health Care System

The patient, the family and friends of the patient, and health care providers must all be aware of the *physical and emotional* impact of any given illness. This is necessary if the patient is to realize optimal benefits from interacting with the health care system. Comprehensive treatment of mind and body helps to: (1) optimize physical functioning; (2) maintain emotional stability and prevent the development of an abnormal illness response; (3) prevent the serious disruption of close relationships with family members and friends; and (4) support the highest level of day-to-day functioning, including professional and social responsibilities.

Many individuals are capable of working through the distressing feelings attending the loss of health. And many medical personnel are attuned to these emotions in a way that permits *collaborative* medical treatment, embodied in Parsons's conceptualization of the "sick role" (see Chapter 9). Effective, humane care is founded on the positive interaction between the patient and the health care provider where both parties have distinct responsibilities for the

143

treatment. In the throes of an illness, the patient abdicates considerable control to caretakers, who willingly accept the patient's dependency until an improvement in clinical status permits more autonomous functioning. This process requires that the patient have a comprehensive intellectual and emotional appreciation of the disease process, and that medical personnel respond with empathy to facilitate an *overall* adjustment to illness. For example, following a stroke that causes partial paralysis, the health care providers should simultaneously guide the physical rehabilitation and help the patient work through the emotional upheaval.

Unfortunately, this quality of medical treatment is often more of an ideal than a reality, because of the nature of the health care delivery system. Issues endemic to the medical world interfere with the biopsychosocial model of treating mind and body, preventing patients from receiving the necessary attention to important psychosocial issues affecting, and affected by, their physical illness. These issues can generally be discussed in the context of the following categories: (1) the structure of the health care system; (2) the medical, or treatment, environment; and (3) the personal interactions of patient and family with health care providers.

The Structure of the Health Care System

The post–World War II era has been a period of remarkable medical advances. The trend toward medical subspecialties, coupled with sophisticated technological achievements, has greatly increased the level of medical expertise available to patients. Unfortunately, one cost of these improvements in medical treatment has been a growing depersonalization in health care, resulting in a general reluctance to treat the patient as a "whole" human being.

Generalist Versus Specialist

The traditional practice of medicine in the United States centered on the family doctor. A single practitioner treated an entire family over the course of their lives, and often into the next generation. The general practitioner's approach was ideally suited to a biopsychosocial approach to medical care. The G.P. or, in the more recent past, the internist, was not just a doctor but also a confidante, an adviser intimately involved in the lives of patients. That era, however, has given way to the current practice of medical care based on separate visits to carefully selected specialists for specific complaints.

Medical education reflects, and indeed fosters, this kind of specialization. Despite many schools' recent attempts to stress humanism and the treatment of the "compleat patient," an emphasis on specialization still pervades medical training. The course of study still subscribes to a cause-and-effect orientation in which medical care is predominantly based on a thorough understanding of the physical aspects of a specific illness, its signs, symptoms, and recommended treatment. This body of knowledge is certainly essential for the effective practice of medicine; however, too great an emphasis on these physical issues causes health care providers to forget to consider the patient as a whole person.

Patients generally receive sympathetic and encouraging support from medical caregivers. However, this interaction often becomes increasingly depersonalized as treatment proceeds, when laboratory tests, hospital charts, and relevant medical articles progressively receive more attention than the patient. Consider the episode involving a woman who had become severely debilitated and disoriented because of her steadily increasing, uncontrollable blood pressure. During the last minutes of her life, with relatives huddled around her bedside, the attending physician attempted to elicit what he considered to be necessary medical data—completely unaware that it was far more important for her family to share in her final moments. This painful illustration of the physician-as-technician is a reminder of how a highly trained specialist could develop such tunnel vision and lose sight of the total patient. This woman had lost her identity and, consequently, her dignity in the morass of the medical world. Defined solely by her pathology, she was not allowed to die in peace, in the comforting presence of her family.

Many patients are reassured by their doctors' very specialized training. However, there is a greater potential for impersonal care with a specialist; the kind of care that fosters the dichotomy between treatment of a particular part of the body and treatment of the total patient. Consulting specialists often see a patient only once or twice, which, by definition, makes them less inclined to form a personal attachment. Instead, the referring physician is left to deal with any psychosocial issues that may arise from the consultation.

The case of William Cunningham illustrates how a medical generalist can successfully attend to the patient's behavior as well as physical problems. Mr. Cunningham, age forty-five, had been feeling tired and sluggish, so he went to his internist for a checkup. His doctor discovered that he was seriously anemic and became concerned that Mr. Cunningham might have an occult, or hidden, cancer, especially since his father had died of colon cancer at a young age. Mr. Cunningham was twice scheduled to undergo a colonoscopy, a definitive diagnostic test. Each time he "suddenly remembered" a business trip that had actually been planned after the test was scheduled. Even though he was concerned about what was wrong, he was ambivalent about finding out, owing to his extreme anxiety that he might be diagnosed with the same illness that had taken his own father. The physician understood why his patient had canceled the procedure. Consequently, he called Mr. Cunningham, rescheduled the test, and insisted that the patient come to the office accompanied by his wife. Preliminary findings indicated a benign polyp. The doctor cautioned him that only the final biopsy results would confirm that favorable diagnosis. When that information was available, he immediately informed the patient, who had already been plagued by the irrational conviction that his biopsy was positive and that he would require immediate hospitalization and surgery. This doctor's attention to his patient's mind and body illustrates good medical practice. Had he not appreciated Mr. Cunningham's overdetermined anxiety about colon cancer, he might have responded differently to his patient's missed appointments. His understanding of his patient's illness dynamics, largely a result of his ongoing relationship with the patient over the years, helped him interpret the significance of his patient's *behavior*, in addition to the significance of his symptom of anemia. William Cunningham's chances of getting lost in the medical system would have greatly increased had he missed two appointments with a busy specialist who had no personal appreciation of him. That physician would probably have responded more slowly—or possibly not at all.

Economic Factors

Economic factors have encouraged the trend toward depersonalized medical care. There is greater pressure on health care providers to implement more rapid treatment, sometimes with fewer resources, because of decreased governmental subsidies, the dictates of their patients' health insurance, and other changes in the economic climate. As a result, most people have shorter hospital stays. Although patients are not summarily discharged in disregard of possible adverse medical consequences, briefer hospitalizations offer them less medical and emotional support and reassurance, and less time for gathering and sharing information. In this way they are given the impression that within the hospital system they really are defined by their physical pathology.

A related trend toward ambulatory surgery has similar effects. Outpatient surgery places a greater burden on family and friends to help patients deal with their feelings about their illness. This is not necessarily a problem for families that cope well with stress. However, even in optimal circumstances, it would probably be easier on everyone to have the added support of hospital personnel, for patients usually rely heavily on these individuals during and after surgical procedures.

Efforts to contain the cost of treatment have led to the formation of HMOs (Health Maintenance Organizations), PPOs (Preferred Provider Organizations), and similar organizations. The arrangements of some of these types of medical practices can make patients feel more like prisoners in the health care system than collaborative players. For example, patients in such plans can be treated only in certain hospitals for certain ailments.

HMOs further depersonalize health care by diffusing the tie between patient and primary care physician. The doctor who treats a patient on a given day may not necessarily be the one seen for previous appointments. At best, this is disruptive to health care; at worst, it can have a detrimental effect on the level of treatment, owing to diffusion of responsibility, poor communication of relevant medical history, and the fact that no single physician gets to know the individual idiosyncracies of a given patient.

These new economic realities in the practice of medicine leave many patients feeling angry and alienated. Their diminished control over how they receive health care, often after having paid considerable insurance premiums, creates a sense of being cheated. This is particularly true if previous care had been more personal, a comparison often made by geriatric patients who remember the "good old days" of the family doctor.

Medical Technology

The medical world offers highly technological tests and procedures. Their benefits are truly revolutionary, but they also insidiously augment the depersonalization within the health care system. If, for example, a patient's CAT scan is normal, the health care providers heave a sigh of relief and inform the patient that "the brain is normal" or that "no masses are in the liver." The good news is certainly welcome, but it doesn't address other feelings about the consequences of the episode of ill health, such as the anxiety experienced before the test, the disruptive effect on the family, or the decline in work performance. Medical personnel tend to give the message that since everything is in order physically, the patient should simply put disturbing emotions aside. That is not a realistic expectation, for the patient may actually need to talk about these feelings with a health care provider. In addition, despite the negative test results, the patient may still not feel physically well. Health providers may minimize, or even disregard, these medical complaints and talk of a "clean bill of health" based on the diagnostic procedure. Health care personnel should tend to the patient's mind, as well as the body, when a test is first recommended, prior to and during the actual procedure, while the results are awaited, and even afterward.

Highly specialized therapeutic interventions, such as coronary bypass surgery, pose similar problems. The procedure can be a success, but the patient can still suffer significant emotional distress if assessed by caretakers exclusively in terms of the operation. The case of Lawrence Coyle provides a good example. Following his successful coronary bypass, Mr. Coyle's eight-year-old daughter joked about buying a heart-lung machine (the life support apparatus used during the procedure) and keeping it at home in case her father "started feeling bad." The well-intentioned joke of a child who feared for her father's welfare began Mr. Coyle's emotional decline to a state of generalized anxiety and intermittent agoraphobia (the fear of going outside). Although the entire procedure had been explained prior to the surgery, this was the first time he truly understood that his survival had been totally dependent on a machine during the operation. Mr. Coyle had always been extremely concerned about maintaining control in his life, but unfortunately his surgeon had no appreciation of this need to be in control. It eventually became the responsibility of his internist, whose long-term relationship with Mr. Coyle provided insight into how he routinely responded to illness, to deal with the postoperative anxiety that was preventing him from returning to a normal life.

Specialized tests or procedures often involve bringing yet another person, the medical technician, into the therapeutic relationship. The individual performing a CAT scan might be well meaning, and even provide useful temporary support to a patient, but chances are good that the only thing he or she knows about that patient is that a test is required in order to rule out significant illness. By bringing more and more people into a patient's life, medical technology dilutes the personal contact of treatment and often increases the potential for disruptive relationships with health care providers.

Recommendations for Negotiating the Health Care System

A primary goal for both patient and family is to attain as much *mastery* as possible over the medical situation. The greater the patient's personal involvement in treatment, the greater the influence he or she can exert over that treatment. Such assertiveness enhances coping. That said, what can be done to minimize those factors inherent in the structure of the health care system that detract from overall medical care? Here are ten suggestions.

1. Whenever possible, a family should try to have one primary care physician, either in an individual practice or in a small group. Get to know the other doctors in a group so that if the regular doctor is unavailable, the family will feel comfortable with his or her replacement, and confident that the patient is receiving optimal care.

2. Whatever the physical complaint, begin treatment with the primary care physician, even if only with a

phone call. The primary care physician has the most comprehensive medical understanding of the patient, based on a long-standing medical relationship. He or she knows the full implications of the patient's physical complaint, has the most accurate appreciation of the patient's emotional makeup, and should be aware of the patient's typical response to illness—whether it be considerable anxiety or depression or denial. The doctor may even be able to determine whether the current complaint is largely due to emotional distress, a physical disorder, or both.

3. If, after contacting the primary care physician, it is necessary to see a specialist, tell the doctor about any personal preferences for a male or female, someone old or young, or someone who will take the time to sit down and talk. Find out which specialists are available and what their individual strengths and weaknesses are. Is one specialist a particularly aggressive physician, more committed to action than watchful waiting? Does he or she prescribe a lot of medication?

    Ask the primary care physician to make personal contact with the referring specialist to communicate important information relevant to the medical case. Or ask the specialist to call the physician to obtain that background information. Just as it is important that medical records get sent to the specialist (and the results of the examination go back to the primary care physician), personal contact between the two doctors is extremely useful in communicating pertinent information about a patient's physical and emotional makeup.

4. When choosing between two specialists, the patient should visit both of them to discuss the medical problem. During each visit, the patient should spell out all concerns, ask all questions, and explain how he or she wants to be treated. This can be couched in terms of "I like my internist because she takes the time to talk to me and answer my questions after she examines

me." It is essential to feel comfortable with the specialist who is ultimately selected.

It helps to have a family member accompany the patient to a specialist. This is particularly useful if the patient had difficulty coping with a previous episode of ill health. A parent, spouse, or friend may anticipate an abnormal illness response and provide needed support that helps the patient manage excessive anxiety, depression, helplessness, or denial brought on by the stress.

Note that consulting a specialist for a new symptom sharply contrasts with the visit to the family doctor. It is likely that the patient is meeting the specialist for the first time. This greatly enhances the possibility that the specialist will look at the patient exclusively in terms of the illness, rather than as a whole person presenting a symptom. Instead of tending to mind and body, the specialist will be highly focused on the physical complaint and more likely to begin an assessment with an established protocol of tests, which further depersonalizes the care. In some cases, the patient might even have the tests before actually talking to the specialist, because office routine dictates that the latter have the test data prior to the appointment. When the test becomes as important—if not more so— than the words, the care is, by definition, too depersonalized.

5. Be economically prepared for the costs of health care. This may sound simplistic, but intelligent planning as a consumer of health care can enormously reduce the stresses attached to coping with illness. Choose health insurance as carefully as possible. A little research can help locate the best policy to provide for special needs (mental health care, liberal provision for cost of medications, etc.) even if no policy is ideal.

6. Investigate the flexibility of insurance coverage. Treatments not usually covered by insurance might be covered under certain circumstances. For example, an

outpatient or surgical procedure might be covered if performed in the hospital when there are certain indications that call for a greater degree of caution, as with a person suffering from unstable heart disease who requires a colonoscopy. If the insurance company requires a letter from the physician in such a case, *do not hesitate* to ask him or her for this documentation. There are no guarantees that the insurance company will agree to pay for the procedure, but trying to obtain coverage helps promote the feeling of being more in control and facilitates coping with the illness.

7. Carefully research an HMO before joining the program. HMOs will often provide the names of some people who would be willing to talk about their experiences with the program. Question current members about their satisfaction or dissatisfaction. In addition, visit the HMO and try to make personal contacts with people who work there. Find out what hospitals patients are referred to for treatment, and verify the reputation of those hospitals.

8. Examine various social service agencies that can provide support for people undergoing medical care. For example, investigate the many publicly funded rehabilitation programs for individuals with chronic illness that do not require acute hospital treatment. When the medical problem is more acute, such as when the patient is recuperating at home from outpatient, ambulatory surgery, the local chapter of the Visiting Nurses Association can provide support.

9. If specialized tests or diagnostic procedures are required, spend time beforehand collecting information. What will the test reveal, and what does that mean regarding the presence or extent of an illness? Ask about possible complications. Can the test result in death or permanent impairment, such as stroke or paralysis? Who will be discussing the test results? When will the results be ready? Will family be kept

fully informed? In addition to eliciting the necessary information, this approach communicates the patient's individual identity to the new people who are providing medical care.

10. Whenever any treatment is being applied—surgery, medications, rehabilitation—always discuss possible adverse reactions. What are the untoward effects of a given operation? What is the fatality rate? How often does a particular medication cause dangerous allergic reactions? Will any mental or physical functions be affected by the drug? Can any treatment cause an additional medical problem due to side effects? The answers to these types of questions must be considered before consenting to any medical treatment.

The Medical Environment

Diverse aspects about the *places* where patients go to be diagnosed, evaluated, and treated affect the way health care is delivered. The appearance of a medical facility, the schedules and routines it follows, the kind of personnel working there, and its values and expectations all have an impact on how patients react to their illnesses. The medical environment may help or hinder the ability to grieve the loss of health, which patients (and families) must achieve if they are to cope successfully with the effects of illness.

The Hospital

Admission to the hospital precipitates strong, ambivalent feelings. On the one hand the patient is reassured by the fact that he or she will be cared for and, it is hoped, cured of a particular health problem. However, fear about the medical condition and the knowledge that there is something potentially or significantly wrong can cause considerable emotional turmoil. Many factors endemic to the hospital routine also heighten this distress. At the very least, confinement in a hospital disrupts the daily routine. It is also an unusual living arrangement: the patient stays in one place all day long for a few or many days, an unnatural confinement that requires a change in personal habits of daily living. Most people find hospitals irritating, frustrating, and embarrassing. The patient is told when—and even what—to eat, when to sleep, what to wear, and how much activity is permitted. There is little privacy in a hospital, and it is difficult for the patient to feel in control of fate when he or she has practically no control over the daily routine. This becomes all the more frustrating when the patient sees other people—family, friends, doctors, nurses, and other personnel—come and go as they please.

Hospital patients repeatedly complain about the *insensitive* environment. It starts at the time of check-in, where the complicated administrative procedure requires a great deal of paperwork. Patients often wonder why they're required to fill out forms and answer a lot of nonmedical questions when they are coming in for physical care. Hospitals tend to be vast physical complexes staffed by large numbers of unknown people. Even though the patient entrusts a most precious possession—the body—to the hospital, frequently he or she feels insignificant, an intruder in this environment. Moreover, there is often the feeling that hospital personnel do not help the patient overcome this feeling. A patient may observe personnel behaving in a very cavalier way toward people who are sick, even gravely ill. The patient has no way of knowing or understanding the desensitization that happens to hospital workers who witness all kinds of illness and, often, death. This routine aspect of a hospital worker's job is foreign, and frightening, to the patient, who may also hear hospital personnel complain about, even criticize, other patients. It's hard to be philosophical about hospital personnel who fail to demonstrate considerable sensitivity and concern *all* the time. But it's important to remember that each patient is merely one of many assigned to these caretakers, who are often stressed by the demands of work. They usually have an appreciation of each patient as an individual—but may not always demonstrate it.

The hospital environment is also *disorienting* to most patients. The strange surroundings can be even more disruptive when someone is in traction and confined to a bed for many weeks. The patient's sleep pattern is often disturbed, either because the patient is continually being awakened at odd hours, by staff or other patients, or simply because of his or her difficulty adjusting to the environment. In addition, many medications interfere with sleep or cause the patient to feel "spacey," which can create even greater insecurity. Hospitalization may cause a major change in a person's social situation, which can be further disorienting. Consider how it would feel for a farmer to wind up in a sophisticated, high-tech medical center; or for the high-powered, fast-paced CEO, accustomed to asserting authority, to take orders from all levels of hospital personnel. With older, or demented people, a phenomenon called "sundowning" can also occur. These individuals rely on external stimuli to reinforce their everyday reality. At home, they can have night lights, television, radio, and easy access to the outside world. The constant input of these kinds of stimuli in recognizable surroundings helps to keep them mentally sharp. When these stimuli are denied them in a hospital, usually at night, they can get easily confused.

For all these reasons, hospitals are frightening, frustrating places. The environment stirs intense feelings in patients that often make it difficult to grieve the loss of health and cope with illness.

Specialized Environments

A special ward in a hospital can be at once reassuring and frightening. Patients in a cardiac intensive care unit know that the staff are experts trained to deal with any emergency that might arise, and that the specialized equipment they need is readily available. On the other hand, patients are aware that they are in the ward because their condition is considered quite serious. Watching and listening to the cardiac monitors, they know that if the cardiogram changes, or if the alarm sounds, something bad may be happening. They see the "crash cart" with its defibrillator (the electric paddles used to shock a heart back to activity) and the images of its use are frightening. Since the mortality rate of patients is higher in the ICU, patients become keenly aware of the number of people who have died, wondering if their own death is imminent.

A renal dialysis unit is a medical environment that provides patients with chronic life support. Obviously, they are reassured by the miracle of this technology, though the realization of just how much they need those machines often stirs fear and resentment. Moreover, though patients appreciate their ongoing relationships with caring, supportive personnel who staff dialysis units, they also recognize their considerable dependence on them. This, too, can foster feelings of resentment.

A neonatal ICU is a very frightening environment for parents and children alike. In the first place, it is often impossible to get a verbal assessment of how the patient feels being hooked up to intricate machinery that restricts movement and sometimes causes pain—though we can speculate about its impact on the child. From the parents' perspective, there is the worry that goes with knowing their child requires such intensive care, despite the reassurance that he or she is getting it. Parents are also usually prevented from physically interacting with their child, stirring feelings that range from deprivation to anger.

Specialized Treatments

Another factor in determining the response to the medical environment is the type of procedure the patient has had or will be having. After open-heart surgery, for example, a certain percentage of patients develop postoperative psychosis. It is not known why this happens—speculation ranges from biologic to psychologic reasons—but the phenomenon is real, and patients must be treated for their psychotic disorientation, as well as for the cardiac condition. Patients who have had bone marrow transplants feel the emotional effects of having undergone such a delicate and specialized procedure, coupled with their subsequent isolation in a sterile, plasticized environment for many weeks with no opportunity for contact with other people.

Methods of Coping While Hospitalized

As discussed in Chapter 4, gathering facts is an important component of coping. Just as that cognitive process is helpful during the diagnostic phase of illness, so too is it a good idea to learn as much as possible about the particular medical environment. For example, tour the institution before being admitted to a hospital. Visit the delivery room, or the dialysis center, or whatever other facilities are relevant. If a specialized test, like a CAT scan, is required, obtain printed material about the procedure. Ask about general details of checking into the hospital, and the specific issues related to hospitalization for the particular illness. What tests will be necessary preoperatively? How are they performed? How long do they take, and when will the results be available? What findings on a test can change the course of treatment, and how? The family should be actively involved in this process, particularly if the patient cannot handle it because of physical symptoms or excessive emotional distress.

Learn about the day-to-day operations of the hospital. What is the routine? What times are meals served? When are usual tests, like drawing blood, done? Must a hospital gown be worn? Which personnel will the patient and family come in contact with? What's the usual length of stay for someone with this illness? How long is the patient expected to be hospitalized?

Having this information makes it possible to work with the staff to schedule at least some of these activities in a way that is comfortable for the patient, and which does not interfere with the staff's routine. For example, if a test is needed that requires no ingestion of food after midnight the previous evening, try to schedule it for the morning even if this means waiting an extra day for the procedure. It is important to remember that the patient—and the family—have some say in how and when things are done in a hospital. A nonemergency admission can be scheduled at a convenient time, such as during an anticipated lull at work. It's good to have family members around to help with various appointments during the hospital stay—to wait with the patient in the X-ray department, or to meet with the dietician when he or she goes over the diet that must be followed upon discharge. A relative can be a "second pair of ears" to help the patient remember what's been said, and can ask questions that might otherwise be forgotten.

One way to diminish the sense of depersonalization or isolation experienced in the hospital is to let family members provide the structure and support needed to feel more in control. They can help the patient maintain some level of activity, even resume some degree of functioning, by bringing to the hospital some work from the office or some family bills to handle, thus giving the patient something other than the illness to focus on. Feeling more in control of the hospital environment will help foster the feeling of being a person who happens to be a patient, rather than exclusively a patient. People with some level of mastery over their situations enhance their ability to cope with the stress.

Family members should enlist support from outside to help them cope. Medical personnel, such as dialysis technicians or physical therapists, can be a source of information and reassurance. The family can develop relationships with these people and try to facilitate supportive relationships between them and the patient. Family friends can help decrease the isolation of a patient who may be too angry or depressed to reach out, or who may see himself or herself only as sick and not capable of attaining the previous level of functioning. Another avenue for families to explore is outside organizations, including social agencies like the Visiting Nurses Association. Support groups are also useful in helping patients—and families—accommodate to the medical environment. Self-help groups for individuals with specific diseases or conditions—such as cancer, post-stroke, heart disease, AIDS—are increasingly widespread and readily accessible.

Asking for and seeking help when it's needed is a form of adaptive coping, and if a family sees that this would help the patient and/or themselves, it is an important option to pursue. The family's active involvement in the treatment helps the patient and provides the family with greater knowledge about the physical and emotional aspects of the illness. The self-awareness and opportunity for family members to work through their feelings help them get through a stressful time. By focusing their energy on work or tasks, the family can avert or minimize abnormal patterns of family interaction during a difficult period.

Interpersonal Relationships with Medical Personnel

The effect of a patient's—and his or her family's—interpersonal relationship with medical personnel cannot be minimized. Even when patient and family are effectively coping with the impact of illness—the patient grieving the loss of health, the family going through a collective grief process and then becoming actively involved in the patient's care—health care personnel can impede this process. These caregivers (doctors, nurses, physical therapists, and others) may do things that interfere with the emotional, and therefore physical, accommodation to illness. This is often unconsciously motivated (but can be deliberate), either in response to a particular patient or as a manifestation of the health care provider's usual psychological distress.

When a person who is ill is having a pathologic response to illness, strong, negative emotions such as anger or depression are not uncommon. Neither is the presence of irritating behaviors, such as an excessive dependency or extreme denial. These emotions and behaviors can be frustrating to the people trying to care for the patient. What is already an "antitherapeutic" situation becomes more so as medical personnel respond "incorrectly" to the patient. Instead of trying to relate in a way that can help the patient grieve the loss of health, medical personnel respond to his or her negative emotions by getting into a struggle with the patient. Antagonism then replaces the collaborative working alliance between patient and caregivers.

Patients exhibiting these behaviors can often irritate medical personnel, who respond by labeling them "high strung," "complainers," or even "phonies," and behave toward them in a critical or condescending way. Individual caregivers delegate more and more treatment responsibilities to other personnel, such as trainees, in a thinly disguised effort to abandon these patients. The caregivers may be unaware of the fact that an abnormal illness response is actually part of the illness. They fail to realize that they are being drawn into a struggle by patients who are unable to grieve the loss of health. Unfortunately, this type of reaction by health care providers helps perpetuate an abnormal illness response.

Some health care providers cannot tolerate the expression of any degree of emotion, whether it be in their professional or personal lives. As a result, they become uncomfortable or displeased when a patient expresses normal feelings of grief, either by talking openly about them or by demonstrating them through behavior, such as refusing a certain test out of anger. The health care provider may overtly or covertly attempt to stifle the patient's feelings and thereby interfere with his or her adaptation to the loss of health. One way of accomplishing this is to focus increasingly, or exclusively, on the patient's physical ailment, and then become irritated when the patient displays what is considered to be excessive emotion. In these situations, it is the health care provider who disrupts the relationship with patients who are actually trying to work though their feelings about illness. The health care provider is sending a clear message that this is inappropriate behavior and should not be done, at least not in his or her presence.

Alternatively, some health care providers respond to patients who are denying their obvious feelings by aggressively trying to get them to abandon their denial. Lacking an accurate understanding of how to help someone grieve the loss of health, they push the patient to see the "reality" of the situation. However, a person can grieve the loss of health only when he or she is *ready* to do so, not before. Relentlessly confronting the patient about feelings may trigger the sensation of being overwhelmed by emotions. The patient may become panicked by these feelings—and grow even more distraught—or flee from medical care in an attempt to escape the emotional turmoil. This confrontational approach is not always motivated by ignorance. It may reflect particular aspects of a health care provider's personality, such as a personal aggressiveness, or a wish to be in control with little sensitivity to the needs of others. Such an individual merely wants to get his or her way with little regard for what is best for the patient.

Some health care providers have their own psychologic conflicts that foster unhealthy, if not adversarial, interactions with patients. In psychiatric terms, this is known as *countertransference*. This concept refers to feelings a psychotherapist has about patients that actually derive from his or her *own* past experiences. One way of understanding this concept is to think about the situation in which we meet someone whom we instantly like or dislike. That reaction is not based on anything substantive, because it occurs before we have any real appreciation of what that person is like. The immediate reaction is actually based on earlier events; the person we are meeting reminds us unconsciously of someone in our past whom we either liked or disliked. In this kind of quick response, the new person bears the brunt—positive or negative—of the feelings we really have for someone else.

The same situation can occur in the relationship between patients and health care personnel. One manifestation is when both patient and doctor have similar personality styles, and they ultimately wind up in conflict with each other. This is most apt to happen when a patient's basic personality is competitive and controlling. That individual is just acting naturally when questioning a doctor's orders, such as the use of a specific medication or a special diet. Most physicians will respond positively to this; they respect the patient's input and may be amenable to changing a prescription from one medication to another. But if the physician in question has a strong need to feel in control of a situation arising from his or her own life experiences, upbringing, and past relationships, it could adversely affect the doctor-patient relationship. Out of a need to be in control, the doctor may simply disregard the patient's input and insist that as a trained professional, he or she knows what's right.

Another countertransference seen in health care providers relates to the terminal course of some cancer patients that reminds them of their own limitations. This, in turn, may provoke a sense of helplessness that is acted out against both patient and family, either by underestimating the patient's retained ability to function or by offering false reassurance in the face of a grave clinical situation. In addition to shaping treatment decisions that may decrease the patient's daily comfort level—for example, excessive use of analgesics and sedatives—this negativistic response may also stir painful emotions such as shame, anger, or guilt in the patient, which will negatively affect all of his or her relationships.

Many health care providers have a healthy predilection toward specific patients, as determined by factors such as age (young versus old) or the course of the illness (acute versus chronic), likes and dislikes that do not usually interfere with treatment. However, as stated previously some medical personnel are plagued by unconscious prejudices that negatively affect a patient's day-to-day care and ability to accommodate the loss of health.

Some Practical Recommendations

1. Patient and family alike must monitor how they feel *and* how medical personnel make them feel. These assessments must be made not only when good news is being communicated, but also when receiving bad news or undergoing as yet inconclusive medical treatment. One sign of a problem in the therapeutic relationship is if the patient or the family *always* have negative feelings—anxiety, anger, depression, or even boredom—when meeting with a particular health care provider. While a negative response to a particular physician can be a component of the emotional response to illness, it is reasonably safe to assume that some kind of problem exists if patient and/or family never are given any reassurance by a particular physician; or don't feel confident about that physician's skills, despite recommendations and reassurances of his or her expertise by medical personnel who are trusted.

   The cause of such problems may be complicated, such as the physician's own feelings intruding on the relationship, or it may be the simple fact that he or she is a bad match for the patient and family. If a patient (or family member) feels this way, it should be discussed openly among the family, so they can compare notes, and brought to the attention of the health care provider in question. That individual may even help the family make a determination whether these feelings will complicate or impede treatment.

   Arlene O'Brien, a forty-seven-year-old advertising executive, was told that she needed to have her left breast removed as a result of cancer. A voracious reader, Ms. O'Brien remembered having recently seen a report on the various treatment options available to breast cancer patients. One of the options discussed at length was a lumpectomy (removal of the lump, with the breast left relatively intact), along with chemotherapy. Since Ms. O'Brien was interested in learning more about this option, she questioned her doctor, only to learn that he was a strong proponent of mastectomies. He stated his belief that a mastectomy was the best method for removing any traces of cancer and told Ms. O'Brien there didn't need to be any further discussion on the matter. She was understandably upset—both with her doctor's manner and with his rigidity and refusal to listen to her. Recognizing that conflict did not bode well for their relationship, she chose another surgeon.

2. When the patient or a family member has negative feelings about the relationship with the doctor, seek a second opinion. This affords the opportunity to hear another person present information about the medical condition, which serves to strengthen cognitive understanding of the situation. The information may corroborate what is already known or may include additional details, such as alternative treatment options.

   Consultation with a second physician also presents the opportunity to compare his or her style of relating and demeanor with that of the first physician. This gives a sense of how accurate the assessment of the first physician was. If, for example, the second doctor says the same things and exhibits the same behavior as the first, there's a chance that the original assessment was incorrect. If, on the other hand, a completely different opinion is formed about the two physicians, the initial judgment was probably right.

   If patient and family are genuinely left confused by two different opinions, there is every reason to seek a third. But "doctor shopping," where a patient frantically searches for the "perfect" doctor, is not recommended. This is often a means of diverting attention from the true medical condition, and often delays definitive treatment.

3. If interpersonal problems arise between patient and caretakers, they must be discussed openly and honestly with these providers. This point cannot be emphasized enough, particularly since many patients and their families feel inhibited about pursuing this course. The doctor-patient relationship is based on mutual trust and respect, with both parties working toward the common goal of improving the patient's health. Anything that interferes with this relationship also interferes with the attainment of that goal. If the patient feels angered by the doctor or physical therapist, or feels he or she has changed and isn't as concerned as before, or if the caregiver *seems* distant when talking about the illness, *discuss these issues with him or her.* That person may have changed in a way that affects interactions, and though that change may have nothing to do with the patient (health care personnel also have personal lives), it has an impact, nevertheless.

When sensing a change in a relationship with an important health care provider, ask if he or she has also noticed some difference. If the answer is yes, follow the logical course of the discussion. Explore together why there has been a change and closely listen to what he or she says. The doctor may have sensed a change in the patient, observing increasing anger as the impact of the illness sinks in. Or circumstances in the doctor's personal life may account for his or her behavior. The doctor may see a decline in the patient and start to act distant to protect against being affected emotionally by any further deterioration. On the other hand, the doctor may see the patient as improving, soon to leave the hospital, and be distancing as a means to avert his or her own sense of loss. Or perhaps the doctor is reacting to a particular family member who has been making the treatment process more difficult.

4. If there is a *particular problem*, discuss it with the appropriate medical personnel. Obviously, no system can ever be perfect; there will always be some negative developments. However, certain issues are reasonable topics for discussion and can usually be resolved easily with a reasonable person. If, for example, after arriving on time, it always takes an hour to be seen in the doctor's office, insist on coming when the staff will be ready. If a treatment, such as physical therapy, is tiring because the therapist appears to be pushing too hard, discuss this with him or her. The patient and family should talk directly to the person involved with a specific issue. If that doesn't resolve the situation, ask the physician to raise the issue with that person. The doctor can also be asked to serve as a mediator or facilitator for discussion when debating the issue directly with the party involved. This is an especially good approach if previous discussion didn't resolve the problem.

5. Remember that it's possible to change doctors and hospitals and to refuse certain tests and medications. In an acute medical situation, control is likely to be minimal, but when the condition is stable, the patient and family have ultimate control. In a situation where the patient simply cannot work out the differences with a doctor, he or she not only is free to leave—but should leave. For example, a person uses an excellent internist but finds the doctor simply too forward. The internist asks probing questions about the patient's personal life, which the latter dodges, but the internist's persistence with the inquiries makes the patient feel increasingly uncomfortable. Despite his or her acknowledged abilities as a physician, the doctor and patient are not going to work well together owing to this fundamental difference in style. It's time to ask for a referral to another doctor. A more serious example concerns the busy practitioner who "just doesn't have time" to

talk with his or her patients or to meet with their families. This type of doctor, who projects an image of being more of a technician than a humanist, will make the patient feel more like an object than a person.

It usually requires a significant disruption in care for a patient to decide to leave a doctor or refuse a recommended treatment. However, patients motivated and intelligent enough to do the proper information gathering are certainly capable of making these types of decisions. Moreover, they should do so when circumstances suggest that such actions will improve the quality of health care.

An episode of illness involves patients and their families in a series of interpersonal relationships with one another and with health care personnel. If these relationships are not handled in a constructive, supportive fashion, it can have serious repercussions on the patient's prognosis and return to functioning. The vast majority of health care providers are empathic and competent people who are doing a difficult job. However, if they do not act in a satisfactory manner, or if there is a specific problem with certain individuals, it is up to the patient and the family to take the initiative in getting what is needed from these people.

12

When Patients Can't Cope

Having difficulty coping with the impact of an illness is not unusual. Whenever this happens, it is imperative that the patient, and/or the family, recognize the situation in order to limit or abolish its detrimental effects. This is the necessary first step toward initiating definitive actions that will facilitate the grief process that normally accompanies illness and thereby enhance the capacity to cope.

Asking the Right Questions

How can a patient and family correctly assess whether they are dealing effectively with an episode of illness? How can they tell if the patient is receiving optimal treatment for the physical problem, if he or she is grieving the loss of health, and if all family members are undergoing the necessary emotional reactions? And how can they determine whether the health care system is helping or impeding the patient's physical and emotional accommodation to ill health?

169

The following questions provide helpful guidelines for resolving these important issues.

1. Do both patient and family feel that they are well-informed about the illness, its treatment, prognosis, long-term effects, and any other relevant issues? Do they feel that they have sufficient factual information to understand the illness intellectually?

2. Does the patient recognize that he or she is experiencing intense, shifting emotions characteristic of the normal grief process? Does the family see that the patient is going through the grief process? Do they understand how an abnormal illness response can relate to the patient's expressions of emotion, such as excessive anger, depression, or denial?

3. If the family observes an abnormal illness response, does this become a topic for open conversation? Do family members come up with a strategy to deal with this situation, such as openly discussing their observations with the patient or enlisting the help of medical personnel to help the patient understand the realities of the situation? Or does the family simply avoid any type of confrontation?

4. Is the family actively involved in the patient's diagnostic evaluation and treatment? Have they made an attempt to find out what the major characteristics of the medical condition are, what support they can offer (both in the short- and the long-term), and what the patient must do? Do they know which decisions have to be made immediately and which ones can wait? Have they taken any part in that decision making?

5. What is the family's emotional response to the patient's illness, both as a group and as individuals? Are they grieving, experiencing the variety of intense feelings that characterize this process? Do they feel that they are in control of their emotions, or that their emotions are controlling them?

6. Is adaptive coping taking place? Is the patient dealing with most of the necessary tasks related to the illness (see Chapter 4), passively listening to health care providers and family members, while taking little, or no, active role in achieving these necessary goals? Are family members having difficulty judging the degree of the patient's adaptive coping? Does the family have sufficient perspective to recognize its own ability to cope? Is the family making decisions according to the advice of medical personnel (for instance, determining whether the patient can be cared for at home)? Are family members speaking openly among themselves and with the patient about the illness? Are they dealing with the limitations imposed on the patient by the illness, such as paralysis or difficulty speaking after a stroke? If the family works with the issues confronting them, discussing and planning for the long-term effects of the patient's illness—financial consequences, further physical decline, increased pain, lack of intimacy with spouse—it is safe to assume that the family is trying to adaptively cope with the illness.

7. Finally, do the patient and family feel like active participants in the medical word, or do they feel like prisoners, passive bystanders unable to affect the patient's treatment? Do they have a collaborative relationship with medical personnel that permits a give-and-take dialogue? Throughout an episode of illness, from the diagnostic workup through the extended course of an illness, both the patient and the family should feel that they can positively influence the various phases of care. There should be adequate and effective communication with health care personnel about the patient's physical condition, the emotional reactions to the illness, all prescribed treatments and medications, and the prognostic realities. The patient and family must take definitive steps with health care personnel when they feel treatment is too mechanical and impersonal.

Overview of Medical Psychotherapy

What if a patient is unable to grieve the loss of health, unable to adjust to the illness? What if this affects emotional health, the family's stability and functioning, treatment, and ultimately the physical condition? If the patient understands that he or she is having difficulty adapting to the illness, or if the situation is recognized by a family member or a health provider, what can be done? In this circumstance, a special psychiatric treatment, called *medical psychotherapy*, is required.

Like other forms of psychotherapy, medical psychotherapy is predominantly a *talking* treatment, though different types of medications—such as antianxiety or antidepressant agents—are sometimes used in conjunction. The treatment is guided by the health care provider's understanding of the patient's illness dynamics. The therapist is usually a psychiatrist, though it can be anyone whom the patient works with and trusts—a family practitioner, obstetrician, nurse, social worker—and who is knowledgeable about the patient's illness dynamics. The therapist explores with the patient, and sometimes the family, the patient's physical and psychosocial response to the illness. Medical psychotherapy consists of focused discussions on various implications of the patient's illness. It can be employed both in crisis situations, during the acute onset of an illness like a heart attack, for example, or in chronic conditions, such as rheumatoid arthritis. In cases of chronic illness, the patient may choose to focus on the psychological impact of an acute flare-up, or may prefer to talk about the emotional effects of steady physical decline, or both.

There are two basic forms of psychotherapy: supportive, and introspective, or exploratory. The basic goal of supportive therapy is to help patients control the intense feelings precipitated by a particular trauma, stress, or inner conflict, so that they are not overwhelmed by those feelings. Supportive psychotherapy, by seeking to preserve an emotional status quo, helps patients contain their emotional distress within previously acceptable limits.

Introspective therapy, on the other hand, attempts to heighten patients' psychological insight by exploring specific emotional conflicts. This treatment requires that patients be guided by the therapist along a more self-analytic path in order to help them work through the conflicting emotions they feel are causing specific symptoms or pathologic behaviors.

Either of these basic orientations may be applied to medical psychotherapy. The health care provider must determine which approach is the most appropriate and effective, based on the individual needs of the patient and the family. One of the determining factors includes the type or extent of trauma affecting someone. Overwhelming stress, such as the diagnosis of a life-threatening medical condition, often requires that the initial treatment be focused on supporting the patient to strengthen his or her psychological defenses. Later, after the patient has regained some emotional equilibrium, the focus can shift to a more exploratory mode where the patient analyzes feelings about the illness in a more introspective manner.

The fundamental psychological health of the patient also determines the appropriate form of medical psychotherapy. Some people generally do not handle stress well and respond much better to support during periods of crisis. However, people who are highly adaptive and flexible in their ability to deal with stress may profit greatly from guided introspection during a crisis period.

Finally, the therapist looks at the maturity of the patient's interpersonal relationships; how appropriately and interdependently the patient interacts with the people in his or her life. A person who is guarded and suspicious is not likely to open up to explore personal feelings with a medical caregiver. That individual would probably respond more positively to a therapist who supports his or her usual means of coping with difficult situations. On the other hand, someone whose life is characterized by open, sharing relationships is better suited to exploratory therapy.

Medical psychotherapy is usually supportive. During the acute period of illness, it is almost always supportive, since this is often the time of maximum stress for both the patient and the family. At this point, no matter how psychologically resilient they are, the patient and family members welcome the added support of health care providers, as they begin to assess and cope with the impact of an illness on the various aspects of each of their lives. Often, this approach at the outset enables them to get beyond the initial shock of illness, so that they can individually and collectively grieve the patient's loss of health. Other patients and their families require continued support during the early stages of an illness in order to adjust to the treatment regimen. This can even continue throughout their treatment and sometimes, if they are unable to achieve an appropriate emotional adjustment, during or after convalescence. In this circumstance, there usually exists some type of pathological illness response because these individuals, for a variety of reasons, are never capable of fully grieving their loss of health.

Introspective medical psychotherapy is appropriate for those patients who are incapable of grieving their loss of health on their own. With professional guidance, they can work through the varied, intense emotions stirred by their disease. Their treatment is actually a grief process facilitated by a health provider.

Medical psychotherapy helps patients get through the crisis by helping them maintain focus on the here-and-now. It helps control unrealistic fears accompanying ill health, such as, "I'll be in the hospital forever," or "I'll never be able to go back to work." Medical psychotherapy also supports overall emotional functioning by helping the patient become more active and less a victim of the circumstances dictated by health. As mastery over the situation is achieved, the patient promotes his or her own adaptive coping. By recognizing that it's possible to utilize psychological defenses that have worked in the past, even if they only allow the patient to be more appropriately dependent on the caretakers, he or she learns to deal effectively with the stress of illness. This enhances self-esteem and, in turn, adaptive coping.

The Various Forms of Medical Psychotherapy

An abnormal illness response can be treated in a variety of clinical formats: individual therapy, couples therapy, family therapy, or group therapy.

Case Study: Stan Slade

Stan Slade is a forty-year-old, twice-divorced musician who has had a heart attack. He was awakened in the middle of the night with severe chest pain, nausea, and shortness of breath. These classic signs of heart disease were in fact familiar to him, for family members had experienced them. However, he resisted seeking medical attention for about twelve hours, attributing his distress to a hiatal hernia that had been asymptomatic for several years. It was only after he developed dizziness and lightheadedness that he called 911 for help. Mr. Slade's feelings about his life-threatening illness suggested that the best therapeutic approach would be a supportive one.

The degree of his denial during the first twenty-four hours following the heart attack was clearly within acceptable limits. However, as Mr. Slade related more of his clinical history to the therapist, the denial began to become more suggestive of an abnormal illness response. He "discounted" his parents' death from heart disease with a rationalization about his father's "gallbladder problem" and was vague about his mother's illness. He avoided a threatening consideration of his genetic heritage. His past experience with hospitals, stemming from his parents' illnesses, drove him "almost crazy because of the nonchalant care . . . the lack of any real personal care." However, he equated his current hospitalization with a vacation and even made the slip of calling the hospital a "hotel." He also minimized a recent episode of angina, a poor prognostic sign shortly after a heart attack, and attributed it to an old hiatal hernia despite the remission of pain with nitroglycerin.

Mr. Slade appeared to be terrified by the early onset of a disease process that had killed both his parents, though he was unable to openly express his fear. Instead, he resorted to a covert request for additional support from his caretakers, saying he'd do "whatever I'm instructed to do." This open-ended willingness was largely based on the reasoning that his only chance for survival was through the nurturing he got from his physicians. He seemed to be struggling between two stances toward his illness, neither of them healthy. On the one hand, he attempted to deny the reality of his heart attack; on the other, he presented himself as a passively compliant patient who sensed the seriousness of his condition and completely abdicated responsibility for his welfare to his physicians.

In an attempt to offer support and minimize Mr. Slade's anxiety, the therapist encouraged his dependence on his doctors—at least in the short term—while gently challenging his denial. However, attempts to help Mr. Slade grieve his loss of health and work through his feelings about his heart disease were futile. He was unwilling to expose himself to those emotions. He maintained this deception by utilizing unhealthy psychological defense mechanisms such as denial, distortion, and passive-dependent behavior while congratulating himself for his "positive mental attitude." During the acute phase of a heart attack, denial is actually associated with a better prognosis; but Mr. Slade was well onto the recuperative path, and he remained pathologically blocked on his emotions. He continued to broadcast clear signals that introspection was intolerable; it provoked extreme anxiety in him. His ability to sustain meaningful relationships was questionable, in light of the fact that he had been married three times, which cast doubts on his ability to maintain an ongoing relationship with his doctor. Furthermore, his treatment goals were somewhat unrealistic; he expected an excellent prognosis despite his intention to return to a full work schedule shortly after discharge. In addition, he probably would continue to smoke.

For all these reasons, Stan Slade definitely required a

supportive type of medical psychotherapy to help him cope with the emotions produced by his illness. By exploiting his "positive mental attitude" toward the "hospital-hotel" and his physicians, the therapist hoped to make him as receptive as possible to observations and suggestions. First, the therapist tried to diminish concerns that because of his family history he was fated to die young of progressive cardiac disease. Second, the positive regard he held for his caretakers was encouraged, even if it promoted denial of his negative feelings toward them, for that course would make him most receptive to their prescribed treatments. Suggestions from a valued physician, like his cardiologist, might then incline him toward a more reasonable convalescence. For example, he might choose a gradual return to a full work load, as an alternative to his planned resumption of full activities, a potentially fatal course.

Couples Therapy

Couples work is required when a patient's abnormal illness response threatens an important relationship, often a marriage. The psychological health of both partners, their usual style of interaction, and the specific losses incurred by the patient as a result of the illness are all factors in determining the focus of the treatment.

Case Study: Richard and Sandra Lewin

Richard Lewin, age sixty, has had diabetes for many years. One effect of the disease has been intermittent impotence. Even though Mr. Lewin and his wife, Sandra, had hitherto coped successfully with restrictions caused by his illness, Mr. Lewin's sexual problems were now causing a growing distance between the two of them. They consulted a therapist, who first determined that their relationship could withstand the open expression of each partner's strong emotions. The therapist then helped each of them ventilate their feelings—his guilt about his intermittent inadequacy, her anger that she was being denied sexual pleasure, and his resentment that she seemed more angry with him than sympathetic to his plight. Helping the Lewins identify and acknowledge these emotions ended their retreat from each other, which had resulted from the inability of each to openly discuss these painful feelings. This instance of couples therapy is an example of the introspective type of medical psychotherapy.

Family Therapy

When the psychological well-being of a family is adversely affected by the illness of one of its members, medical psychotherapy can often facilitate the family's accommodation to that illness. This is commonly seen when an elderly parent becomes sick. A middle-age man, for example, may become excessively involved in his father's medical treatment, to the degree that he neglects his own family and work responsibilities. He may be so preoccupied with his father's health that he intrudes on the treatment, pestering doctors with the details of his father's symptoms or giving opinions on experimental treatments he has read about. The tension within the son may produce similar tension within his own family and possibly disrupt its normal functioning. In these circumstances, medical psychotherapy often involves the whole family, since everyone is paying some emotional price because of illness in an elder member.

Family-oriented medical psychotherapy may actually be part of a patient's overall treatment regimen. This is often one component in the treatment of eating disorders, such as anorexia nervosa. Many people believe that family interactions cause, contribute to, or aggravate the symptoms of an anorectic patient. Consequently, some clinicians employ family therapy as a basic component of the patient's treatment. This approach is also utilized with asthmatic children. These patients—and their parents—often experience persistent feelings of anxiety or helplessness owing to the unpredictability of the attacks and their frightening nature: an inability to breathe characterizes each episode. In addition to providing reassurance to their child, parents may also communicate their anxiety, which can affect the acute and ongoing course of the illness. A vicious cycle may become established, where the child develops early symptoms of an attack, increasing the parents' anxiety, which is then communicated back to the child. This may aggravate the child's tension, resulting in such physiologic reactions as rapid breathing, which can ultimately precipitate a full-blown asthma attack. These types of emotional interactions are addressed in family-oriented medical psychotherapy, which can be either supportive or introspective, depending on the psychological health of a particular family.

Group Therapy

Group therapy is a form of treatment in which a number of patients assemble and discuss their psychological problems. These may be general issues, like depression or unsatisfactory personal relationships, or focused on more specific areas, such as marital problems or phobic symptoms. Groups are usually conducted by a leader, the defined therapist, who helps guide and facilitate the discussion. However, the basic responsibility for the group's work falls on its members, who benefit in several ways from their interaction. One benefit is information sharing, a cognitive function of groups that helps educate members. Patients may learn that distressing symptoms are actually common to their problem. For example, an individual might discover that a decreased sexual drive is common with depression. Another benefit is the comfort and confidence people usually derive from sharing their feelings with others. The generalized acceptance of emotional expression by groups helps decrease a person's sense of isolation and separation from others in his or her life, feelings that often accompany emotional difficulties. Groups also allow people to discuss important issues in their lives in *displacement,* that is, in a nonthreatening environment, apart from the actual context of their problems. For example, a man unable to express certain feelings toward his wife has the opportunity to discuss these issues openly with others, observe their reactions, and then become comfortable enough to be more direct with his wife. The group setting affords the opportunity to try things out before broaching the issues with the people in the patient's life.

In light of the positive benefits of group interaction, this form of treatment is well suited for medical psychotherapy. Self-help groups provide mutual support for people with the same or similar illnesses, affording them the opportunity to discuss common medical experiences. Throughout the country, there are groups for diabetics, heart attack victims, people who have required amputations, women who have had mastectomies, and AIDS patients. Self-help groups give these individuals a forum to share their feelings of anger, shame, embarrassment, depression, and distorted self-images due to their perception of "being different." They also discuss specific issues, such as fears of recurrent attacks, and feelings about changing their daily routines, diets, or work schedules.

Group work has been advocated as part of the treatment of certain illnesses, usually those considered to be "psychosomatic," where emotions play a significant part in the onset or recurrence of symptoms. Migraine headaches and asthma are two examples that fall into this category. Patients learn about the emotional circumstances that may be involved in the onset of an attack. As part of a self-discovery process, they may also look at why they place themselves in situations that might trigger an attack. They discuss ways to avoid those circumstances, how to abort an attack, or how to minimize its effects. They may also explore feelings that are associated with an attack and study the relationship between these emotions and their physical symptoms.

Patients with terminal illness face many emotional issues that can be effectively addressed in a group situation.

Dying is extremely difficult to contemplate let alone discuss openly with those close to you. Some patients are so overwhelmed by impending death that they simply deny it, and their families often perpetuate the myth. The intention is to "make things easier" by not discussing the awful reality, but a conspiracy of silence usually aggravates the already intense emotional distress. This may be manifested by a distancing among the family members, causing an increasingly desperate isolation from one another. Medical psychotherapy in a group setting is ideally suited to address this situation. It usually combines the supportive and introspective approach, in which patients provide one another with reassurance and support, then collectively explore and work through the feelings they have concerning their mortality. Without an opportunity to ventilate these emotions, patients often retreat from their day-to-day world and die a lonely death.

Comprehensive Medical Psychotherapy

Two general points should be made concerning the practice of medical psychotherapy. First, the idiosyncratic intricacies of a patient's response to illness often require that various forms of medical psychotherapy be used in combination. For example, a woman may deny the seriousness of her symptoms to her spouse because she "doesn't want to worry him," while being very open with work colleagues or another family member. She may request a great deal of support from these other individuals, which they may find burdensome, and simultaneously minimize obvious symptoms to her physicians out of fear that if she gave an accurate medical history, the dreaded diagnosis of multiple sclerosis would be confirmed. This particular response to illness is quite complex. Couples work is recommended to help the woman share her true feelings with her husband. As her denial diminishes, and the underlying emotions begin to emerge, she may develop an abnormal illness response that requires long-term individual treatment. By utilizing a combination of these different forms of medical psychotherapy, health providers can effect a comprehensive treatment that targets the distinctive needs of both patient and family.

Second, medical psychotherapy has been discussed within the context of a single episode of ill health. However, most illness is chronic, and its elongated time course has implications for the practice of this specialized form of psychotherapy. The onset of a long-term illness may so overwhelm an individual that he or she desperately requires supportive treatment at that time. Some patients require that approach throughout the many years of their disease. On the other hand, some people's coping mechanisms may change over the course of a prolonged illness to the point that they can weather on their own the emotional distress caused by exacerbation of their illness. This may reflect the fact that the initial support gave them a sense of mastery over their illness, which in turn promoted the acquisition of new coping mechanisms, and sufficiently increased their self-esteem so they were better able to handle the next episode of ill health. If a patient possesses a more realistic view of his or her illness, fearful fantasies can, over time, be replaced with the reality of symptomatic relief, loving support from family and friends, and a level of functioning that affords some sense of control over the illness regardless of how chronic it may become. Minimizing the emotional turmoil that accompanies each bout with the disease may even render future medical psychotherapy unnecessary.

All medical illness produces emotional responses that form an integral part of the disease process. The preceding pages have highlighted the following fundamental points concerning this interrelationship.

1. Illness is a biopsychosocial experience, affecting and affected by the mind, the body, and the diverse aspects of the social environment.

2. Everyone has a distinctive response to an episode of

ill health that is determined by idiosyncratic illness dynamics.

3. Illness precipitates a grief process, a normal emotional adjustment to the loss of health. By working through the varied feelings accompanying illness, the patient is able to gain a necessary emotional perspective on this stressful period.

4. By diminishing emotional turmoil, grieving facilitates rational decision making by the patient and the family, a hallmark of adaptive coping.

5. The inability to grieve effectively the loss of health precipitates a pathologic illness response. In this circumstance, the patient gets stuck in one of the phases of normal grief and expresses the emotion that characterizes that stage. These abnormal illness responses have a detrimental effect on the patient's physical, as well as emotional, well-being.

6. Just as the patient has to accommodate to the particular loss of health, so does the family, both as an aggregate of individuals and as a unit. Families may effectively accommodate to a member's illness or themselves experience a pathological response.

Most patients and families successfully adjust to the loss of health. Those unable to negotiate the accompanying emotional turmoil suffer abnormal illness responses. For medical care to be effective, both medical personnel and the patient's family must understand what a particular disease means to a particular patient at a particular time in life. This requires a full understanding of his or her illness dynamics, which define a distinctive biopsychosocial environment that guides relatives and health care providers to the specific psychological needs to be addressed during the course of treatment. If this approach fails to abort an abnormal illness response, mental health personnel can offer more focused attention through medical psychotherapy, a psychiatric intervention also based on the patient's illness dynamics. This overall biopsycho-social approach is the only acceptable medical model, a collaborative effort by the patient, family, and health care personnel that is based on openness, empathy, and trust, and that treats the patient as a human being, as opposed to someone defined exclusively by the nature of the illness.

References

Adsett, C., and J. Bruhn. 1968. Short-term group psychotherapy for myocardial infarction patients and their
wives. *Journal of the Canadian Medical Association* 99:
577–81.

Amkraut, A., and G. Solomon. 1974. From the symbolic
stimulus to the pathophysiologic response: immune
mechanisms. *International Journal of Psychiatry* 5:541–
63.

Balint, M. 1957. *The doctor, his patient and the illness*. New
York: International Universities Press.

Bilodeau, C., and T. Hackett. 1971. Issues raised in a group
setting by patients recovering from myocardial infarction. *American Journal of Psychiatry* 128:73–78.

Binger, C., A. Alblin, R. Feuerstein, J. Kushner, S. Zoger,
and C. Nikkelson. 1969. Childhood leukemia: emotional
impact on patient and family. *New England Journal of
Medicine* 280:414–18.

Borden, W. 1962. Psychological aspects of a stroke: patient
and family. *Annals of Internal Medicine* 57:689–92.

Bowen, M. 1966. The use of family theory in clinical practice. *Comprehensive Psychiatry* 7:345–74.

———. 1971. Family therapy and family group therapy. In *Comprehensive Group Psychotherapy*, ed. H. Kaplan and B. Sadock. New York: Williams and Wilkins.

Brown, J., and G. Stoudemire. 1983. Normal and pathological grief. *Journal of the American Medical Association* 250(3):378–82.

Engel, G. 1968. A life-setting conducive to illness: the giving-up/given-up complex. *Annals of Internal Medicine* 69:293–98.

———. 1971. Sudden and rapid death during psychological stress. *Annals of Internal Medicine* 74:771–82.

———. 1977. The need for a new medical model: a challenge for biomedicine. *Science* 196:129–36.

———. 1980. The clinical application of the biopsychosocial model. *American Journal of Psychiatry* 137:535–44.

Frank, J. 1961. *Persuasion and healing*. Baltimore: Johns Hopkins University Press.

Greene, W., S. Goldstein, and A. Moss. 1972. Psychosocial aspects of sudden death. *Archives of Internal Medicine* 129:725–31.

Groves, J. 1978. Taking care of the hateful patient. *New England Journal of Medicine* 298:883–87.

Henry, J. 1975. The induction of acute and chronic cardiovascular disease in animals by psychosocial stimulation. *International Journal of Psychiatry* 6:147–58.

Kahana, R., and G. Bibring. 1964. Personality types in medical management. In *Psychiatry and medical practice in a general hospital*, ed. N. Zinberg, 108–23. New York: International Universities Press.

Klerman, G. 1981. Depression in the medically ill. *Psychiatric Clinics of North America* 4(2):301–18.

Lindemann, E. 1944. Symptomatology and management of acute grief. *American Journal of Psychiatry* 101:141–46.

Lipwoski, Z. 1970. Physical illness, the individual and the coping process. *International Journal of Psychiatry* 1:91–102.

———. 1975. Psychiatry of somatic disease: epidemiology,

pathogenesis, classification. *Comprehensive Psychiatry* 16:105–24.

Livsey, C. 1972. Physical illness and family dynamics. *Advanced Psychosomatic Medicine* 8:237–51.

Lown, B., R. Verrier, and S. Rabinowitz. 1977. Neural and psychologic mechanisms and the problem of sudden cardiac death. *American Journal of Cardiology* 39: 890–902.

Moos, R., and J. Schaefer. 1984. The crisis of physical illness: an overview and conceptual approach. In *Coping with Physical Illness. 2: New Perspectives*, ed. R. Moos, 3–26. New York: Plenum.

Parsons, T. 1951. *The social system.* Glencoe, Ill.: Free Press.

Rioch, M. 1970. The work of Wilfred Bion on groups. *Psychiatry* 33:56–66.

Rodin, G., and K. Voshart. 1986. Depression in the medically ill: overview. *American Journal of Psychiatry* 143:696–705.

Rogers, M., D. Dubey, and P. Reich. 1979. The influence of the psyche and the brain on immunity and disease susceptibility: a critical review. *Psychosomatic Medicine* 41:147–64.

Rosman, B., S. Minuchin, and R. Leibman. Family lunch session: an introduction to family therapy in anorexia nervosa. 1975. *American Journal of Orthopsychiatry* 45:846–53.

Schindler, B. 1985. Stress, affective disorders, and immune function. *Medical Clinics of North America* 69:585–97.

Slaby, A., and A. Glicksman. 1985. *Adapting to Life-Threatening Illness.* New York: Praeger.

Spiegel, D. 1979. Psychological support for women with metastatic carcinoma. *Psychosomatics* 20:780–87.

Spitz, R. 1945. Hospitalism: an inquiry into the genesis of psychiatric conditions in early childhood. *Psychoanalytic Study of the Child* 1:53–74.

Stein, A. 1971. Group therapy with psychosomatically ill patients. *Comprehensive group psychotherapy*, ed. H. Kaplan, and B. Sadock. Baltimore: Williams and Wilkins.

Yalom, I., and C. Greaves. 1977. Group therapy with the terminally ill. *American Journal of Psychiatry* 134:396–400.

Zola, I. 1963. Socio-cultural factors in the seeking of medical aid: a progress report. *Transcultural Psychiatric Research* 14:62–65.

Index

Abnormal group process, 132–35

Abnormal illness response, 143, 161, 170, 181, 183
treatment of, 175–82

Acceptance, 37, 38, 39, 123

Acceptance/resolution stage, 33–34, 41, 64, 67, 127
family, 130

Action, 133

Adaptive coping/response, 22, 34, 47, 52–53, 54, 58–59, 160, 171, 174, 183
anxiety as, 74, 82
denial as, 62
family, 56–58
regression as, 103, 105

Adjustment to treatment outcome (phase), 127–30

Age (stage), 23

Anger, 3, 7, 32, 45, 46, 170

in dependency response, 112–13

in family response process, 123, 126

targets of, 32, 86–89

Anger response, 84–93

Anger stage 31–32, 40, 41, 42, 83, 88

Anxiety, 3, 4, 7, 45, 46
pathologic, 25, 73, 74–75, 82

Anxiety response, 72–83

Asthma, 178–79, 180

Autonomous functioning/autonomy, 41, 43, 47, 49, 54, 88, 104

Behavior, 34, 96, 120
See also Characteristic behaviors

Belief systems, 27

189